COLOR ATLAS OF
DISEASES AND DISORDERS OF CATTLE

Commissioning Editor: Robert Edwards
Development Editor: Veronika Watkins
Project Manager: Nancy Arnott
Designer/Design Direction: Charles Gray
Illustration Manager: Merlyn Harvey

COLOR ATLAS OF
DISEASES AND DISORDERS OF CATTLE

THIRD EDITION

Roger W. Blowey BSc BVSc FRCVS FRAgS

Wood Veterinary Group
Gloucester
England

A. David Weaver BSc DR MED VET PHD FRCVS

Bearsden   Emeritus Professor
Glasgow   College of Veterinary Medicine
Scotland   University of Missouri
            Columbia, Missouri
            USA

Foreword by
Douglas C. Blood

MOSBY
ELSEVIER

Edinburgh   London   New York   Oxford   Philadelphia   St Louis   Sydney   Toronto 2011

First edition © RW Blowey and AD Weaver, 1991
Second edition © 2003, Elsevier Science Limited. All rights reserved.
Third edition © 2011, Elsevier Ltd. All right reserved.

ISBN 978-0-7234-3778-9

British Library Cataloguing in Publication Data
A catalogue record for this book is available from the British Library

Library of Congress Cataloging in Publication Data
A catalog record for this book is available from the Library of Congress

Notices
Knowledge and best practice in this field are constantly changing. As new research and experience broaden our understanding, changes in research methods, professional practices, or medical treatment may become necessary.

Practitioners and researchers must always rely on their own experience and knowledge in evaluating and using any information, methods, compounds, or experiments described herein. In using such information or methods they should be mindful of their own safety and the safety of others, including parties for whom they have a professional responsibility.

With respect to any drug or pharmaceutical products identified, readers are advised to check the most current information provided (i) on procedures featured or (ii) by the manufacturer of each product to be administered, to verify the recommended dose or formula, the method and duration of administration, and contraindications. It is the responsibility of practitioners, relying on their own experience and knowledge of their patients, to make diagnoses, to determine dosages and the best treatment for each individual patient, and to take all appropriate safety precautions.

To the fullest extent of the law, neither the Publisher nor the authors, contributors, or editors, assume any liability for any injury and/or damage to persons or property as a matter of products liability, negligence or otherwise, or from any use or operation of any methods, products, instructions, or ideas contained in the material herein.

ELSEVIER

www.elsevierhealth.com

Working together to grow
libraries in developing countries

www.elsevier.com | www.bookaid.org | www.sabre.org

ELSEVIER   BOOK AID International   Sabre Foundation

The publisher's policy is to use paper manufactured from sustainable forests

Transferred to Digital Printing, 2016

Contents

Contents

Foreword to the First Edition

Textbooks dealing with diseases of cattle have never been good sources of photographic illustrations. They have either omitted pictures altogether or included a collection of disastrous black and white photographs of very poor quality. When I heard that Wolfe were to supplement their excellent collection of colour atlases with one dealing with cattle diseases it was obvious that future books would not feel obliged to add to the existing pictorial indiscretions. This was especially so because my colleagues Roger Blowey in the UK and David Weaver in the USA were bovine clinicians of long and wide experience covering two continents.

The need for these illustrations is obvious. For students at all stages in their careers, good colour pictures can add enormously to their understanding and ability to recognise individual diseases. In recognition of this, most clinical teachers accumulate their own colour transparencies. On several occasions I have looked at my own collection with a speculative eye, but discarded the idea because, like most amateur photographs, they lack the quality that an atlas demands. Most importantly they must illustrate the clinical signs by which the particular disease is recognised. There is no point in a photograph of a thin cow with its head hung down to illustrate tuberculosis, acetonaemia or cobalt deficiency, or a dozen other diseases. What are needed are photographs containing explicit details of specific signs. The photographs also need to be models of photographic artistry, well lit, well composed, with good contrast. Roger Blowey and David Weaver have, for their part, ensured that the photographs are truly illustrative and educational, and that the captions point up the salient features of each illustration in the minimum number of well chosen words.

Many authors, including myself, must have contemplated this task because of its potentially enormous value to veterinary medicine. I congratulate Wolfe and the authors on their courage and perseverance in going ahead and getting it done.

1991
Douglas C. Blood
Professor Emeritus, School of Veterinary Science, University of Melbourne

Preface to the First Edition

For centuries cattle have been the major species for meat and milk production, and in some countries they also serve an additional role as draught animals. Disease, leading to suboptimal production or death, can have a major economic effect on a community reliant on cattle. This atlas attempts to illustrate the clinical features of over 360 conditions. These range from minor problems, such as necrosis caused by tail bands (used for identification purposes), to major infectious diseases, such as foot-and-mouth and rinderpest, which can wreak havoc when introduced into countries and areas previously free of infection. In endemic areas, which all too often include developing countries short of natural resources, they can be a constant source of serious economic loss.

To emphasise the worldwide scope of cattle disease, we have deliberately sought illustrations from many countries. Over one hundred contributors (acknowledged elsewhere) have graphically given this atlas a truly global perspective. Examples come from all five continents: the Americas, Africa, Asia, Europe and Australasia.

Wherever possible, we have tried to illustrate characteristic features of disorders. This has involved the use of a substantial number of internal views of animals. Thus, while the integumentary chapter comprises almost exclusively external views, the respiratory and circulatory sections inevitably contain much more gross pathology. Where single characteristic features do not exist, we have attempted to show typically severe examples of the conditions. Some are difficult to demonstrate in still photography, and this is particularly true of nervous diseases, where the text has been expanded to include behavioural changes.

Each chapter has a brief introductory outline followed, where appropriate, by a grouping of related conditions. No attempt has been made to consider treatment or management of specific conditions, as the atlas is designed to be used alongside standard textbooks. The major emphasis is on the diagnosis and differential diagnosis of conditions, based on visual examination. This aim has been followed with the likely readership in mind: the veterinarian in practice or government service, veterinary students, livestock producers, and agricultural and science students.

We have deliberately excluded microscopic, histopathological and cytological illustrations, since space precludes the large range of illustrations that would have been necessary. Our purpose is to make the atlas comprehensive over the range of international diseases in terms of gross features. In presenting this first attempt at a comprehensive world atlas of cattle diseases, the authors appreciate that some areas may not be covered sufficiently. We welcome suggestions and submissions for improvements to a second edition. We hope that the use of this book will aid and improve the diagnosis of cattle diseases, so permitting the earlier application of appropriate treatment and control measures. We would feel amply rewarded if the atlas helped to reduce both the substantial economic losses and the unnecessary pain and discomfort endured by cattle affected by the many health problems that hinder optimal productivity.

1991   Roger W. Blowey, Gloucester, England
A. David Weaver, Columbia, Missouri, USA

Preface to the Third Edition

The third edition of this atlas follows several reprints and six translations—into Chinese, Danish, French, Japanese, Polish and Spanish—of the previous editions. On the advice of the publisher, American spelling has again been adopted.

Comments in the preface to the second edition have been incorporated into this text to avoid needless repetition. To do justice to the advances in cattle medicine over the last years, which has seen several new diseases assume regional or worldwide importance, the number of illustrations has again been substantially increased (first edition: 732; second edition: 752; third edition: 848), retaining this atlas as one of the major publications in the field of the diagnosis and control of bovine conditions and diseases. In this edition captions have been added to the illustrations for easier orientation of the text.

Among the topics, new or further expanded and illustrated are congenital vertebral malformation, erythropoietic porphyria, and protoporphyria (Chapter 1); bovine neonatal pancytopenia or "bleeding calf syndrome" and incarcerated umbilical hernia (Chapter 2); besnoitiosis, tail sequestrum, and fractured ribs (Chapter 3); abomasal impaction, and jejunal hemorrhage syndrome (Chapter 4); tuberculosis (Chapter 5); cardiac tamponade from tire wire (Chapter 6); digital dermatitis, and crushed tail head (Chapter 7); BVD/MD retinopathy (Chapter 8); fatty liver syndrome (Chapter 9); persistent preputial frenulum (Chapter 10); ischemic teat necrosis (Chapter 11); and botulism (Chapter 12).

Major revisions have been made to three important infectious diseases, namely foot-and-mouth disease, bluetongue, and bovine spongiform encephalopathy (BSE). The advice on management of many diseases and disorders has been revised and expanded, as have the important differential diagnosis sections.

We have again avoided making specific recommendations on drug dosages because product availability and permissible usage varies enormously from country to country, and new products frequently enter the market.

Our warmest thanks go to our many veterinary colleagues who kept a camera in the car or truck ("just in case") and were therefore in a position to supply new material for this edition. As always, thanks go to my (R.B.) clients who, over the years, have been happy for me to stop and take pictures. Drs. Simon Bouisset (France), Enrico Chiavassa (Italy) and John Sproat (Scotland) and several DVMs in the United States of America (responding to the American Association of Bovine Practitioners "grapevine") were particularly generous donors of images and pertinent clinical case histories.

All aspects of animal welfare have assumed increased importance over the last ten to fifteen years. Undoubtedly, disease is a major cause of adverse welfare in our livestock industry, and its improved control will considerably benefit both producers and their stock. This third edition is again directed worldwide towards veterinarians working in all fields of cattle medicine, including diagnostic laboratories, to veterinary and agricultural students, and to livestock producers, whether they are scraping a marginal existence from an unfavorable terrain or are managers of large-scale dairy or feedlot units. We trust the third edition continues to be useful and its widespread application will give us our reward from its production.

April 2010

Roger W. Blowey, Gloucester, England
A. David Weaver, Bearsden, Glasgow, Scotland

Acknowledgments

We are very grateful to our many colleagues (deceased marked[†]) throughout the world who have generously allowed us access to, and use of, their transparencies and have often spent a considerable amount of time selecting them for us. Their help has been invaluable.

Material was supplied by: Mr. J.R.D. Allison, Beechams Animal Health, Brentford, England, 11.40. Prof. S. van Amstel, University of Pretoria, South Africa, 12.31, 12.32. Dr. E.C. Anderson, Animal Virus Research Institute, Pirbright, England, 12.10–12.15. Dr. A.H. Andrews, Royal Veterinary College, England, 3.24, 4.59. Prof. J. Armour, Glasgow University Veterinary Hospital, Scotland, 4.22. E. Sarah Aizlewood, Lanark, Scotland, 5.28, 6.3, 9.8, 12.22. Mr. I.D. Baker, Aylesbury, England, 4.102, 10.56. †Dr. K.C. Barnett, Animal Health Trust, Newmarket, England, 8.5, 8.7. Dr. Simon Bouisset, Colomiers, France, 7.106, 9.19, 9.20, 12.36, 12.68. Dr. Matthew Breed, Clemson University, South Carolina, USA, 4.84. Dr. A. Bridi, MSD Research Laboratories, São Paulo, Brazil, 3.52, 3.54, 3.56, 3.57. Mr. G.L. Caldow, Scottish Agricultural College VSD, St Boswells, Scotland, 2.34–2.36, 3.77, 5.14, 5.15, 10.92, 12.26, 12.27. Dr. W.F. Cates, Western College of Veterinary Medicine, Saskatoon, Canada, 10.38. Dr. Enrico Chiavassa, Cavallermaggiore, Italy, 1.18, 1.19, 2.9, 2.30, 2.50, 4.82, 4.104, 10.57, 10.66. Dr. J.E. Collins, University of Minnesota, USA, 2.17, 2.18. Dr. K. Collins, University of Missouri-Columbia, USA, 8.42. Dr. B.S. Cooper, Massey University, New Zealand, 8.20. Dr. Herder Cortes, Portugal, 3.34. Dr. R.P. Cowart, University of Missouri-Columbia, USA, 1.1. Dr. V. Cox, University of Minnesota, USA, 7.80, 7.82, 7.142. †Mr. M.P. Cranwell, MAFF VI Centre, Exeter, England, 13.6*. Dr. S.M. Crispin, University of Bristol, England, 8.1, 8.3, 8.12, 8.32. †Dr. J.S.E. David, University of Bristol, England, 7.85, 10.39, 10.40, 10.42–10.44, 10.46, 10.47, 10.49–10.53. Drs. J. Debont and J. Vercruysse, Rijksuniversiteit te Gent, Belgium, 4.97. Prof. A. De Moor, Rijksuniversiteit te Gent, Belgium, 1.17, 7.103, 7.153. Dept. of Surgery (Prof. J. Kottman), Veterinary Faculty, Brno, Czech Republic, 7.131, 7.147. Dept. of Veterinary Pathobiology, University of Missouri-Columbia, USA, 1.25, 1.27, 2.21, 2.32, 4.50, 4.58, 4.67, 4.90, 5.5, 5.25, 5.29, 7.115, 9.26, 9.28, 10.3, 10.4, 10.33, 13.7. GD Deventer, Netherlands 12.82. Dr. Daan Dercksen, Animal Health, Deventer, Netherlands, 1.2, 12.16. Prof. G. Dirksen, Medizinische Tierklinik II, Universität München, Germany, 13.6. Prof. J. Döbereiner and Dr. C.H. Tokarnia, Embrapa-UAPNPSA, Rio de Janeiro, Brazil, 2.51, 7.164, 7.165, 7.170, 7.174, 9.32, 13.5, 13.14, 13.15, 13.17, 13.18, 13.24. Dr. A.I. Donaldson, Animal Virus Research Institute, Pirbright, England, 12.4, 12.5, 12.6, 12.7. Dr. S.H. Done, VLA, Weybridge, England, 5.18–5.20*. Dr. J. van Donkersgoed, Western College of Veterinary Medicine, Saskatoon, Canada, 8.11. Mr. R.M. Edelsten, CTVM, Edinburgh, Scotland, 2.12, 3.30, 8.29, 12.29. Dr. N. Evans, Pfizer Animal Health, New York, USA, 5.27. Prof. Fan Pu, Jiangxi Agricultural University, People's Republic of China, 13.34. Prof. J. Ferguson, Western College of Veterinary Medicine, Canada, 7.122, 7.143. Mr. A.B. Forbes, MSD Agvet, Hoddesdon, England, 3.29, 3.50. Mr. J. Gallagher, MAFF VI Centre, Exeter, England, 4.6, 4.7, 7.155, 7.160, 7.167, 7.171, 7.172, 9.17, 9.18, 10.90, 12.77*. Dr. J.H. Geurink, Centre for Agrobiological Research, Wageningen, Netherlands, 13.27, 13.28. Dr. E. Paul Gibbs, University of Florida, USA, 4.2, 4.3, 5.1, 5.6, 5.7, 5.16, 9.35, 11.18–11.28. Mr. P.A. Gilbert-Green, Harare, Zimbabwe, 12.24. Dr. N. Gollnick, Veterinary Faculty, Weihenstephan, Munich, Germany, 3.35, 3.36. Dr. H. Gosser, University of Missouri-Columbia, USA, 4.99, 13.10–13.12. †Dr. W.T.R. Grimshaw, Pfizer Central Research, Sandwich, England, 1.31, 4.41, 4.92, 10.2, 12.76, 12.77, 13.1, 13.2, 13.4. Dr. S.C. Groom, Alberta Agriculture, Canada, 9.29. †Prof. E. Grunert, Clinic of Gynaecology and Obstetrics of Cattle, Tierärztliche Hochschule Hannover, Germany, 10.45. Dr. Jon Gudmundson, Western College of Veterinary Medicine, Saskatoon, Canada, 4.37, 5.31, 5.33, 7.163, 8.22. Mr. S.D. Gunn, Penmellyn Veterinary Group, St Columb, England, 9.41. Mr. David Hadrill, Brighton, England, 12.25. Dr. S.K. Hargreaves, Director of Veterinary Services, Harare, Zimbabwe, 12.2, 12.46, 12.48, 12.63, 13.13. Mr. David Harwood, VLA Itchen Abbas, Winchester, England, 4.68*. Prof. M. Hataya, Tokyo, Japan, 1.11, 7.36. †Prof. C.F.B. Hofmeyr, Pretoria, South Africa, 10.32. Mr. A. Holliman, VI Centre, Penrith, England, 1.35, 2.52, 13.33*. Mr. A.R. Hopkins, Tiverton, England, 10.17, 10.83. Mr. A.G. Hunter, CTVM, Edinburgh, Scotland, 12.61. Mr. Richard Irvine and Dr. Hal Thompson, Veterinary Faculty, University of Glasgow, Scotland, 1.5, 2.10, 2.53, 2.54, 4.43, 4.87, 6.3, 7.83. Dr. P.G.G. Jackson, University of Cambridge, England, 13.30. Dr. L.F. James, USDA Agricultural Research Service, Logan, USA, 13.19. Mr. P.G.H. Jones, European Medicines Evaluation Agency, England, 4.23, 5.26. Prof. Peter Jubb, University of Melbourne, Australia, 7.166. Prof. R. Kahrs, University of Missouri-Columbia, USA, 4.2, 5.1, 5.6. Mr. J.M. Kelly, University of Edinburgh, Scotland, 9.7.

Mr. D.C. Knottenbelt, University of Liverpool, England, 3.82, 8.8, 9.16, 10.30. Dr. R. Kuiper, State University of Utrecht, Netherlands, 3.46, 4.69, 4.70. Dr. A. Lange, University of Pretoria, South Africa, 12.52, 12.53. Dr. E. van Leeuwen, Deventer, Netherlands, 12.17. Dr. L. Logan-Henfrey, International Laboratory for Research on Animal Diseases, Kenya, 12.49–12.51. †Mr. A. MacKellar, Tavistock, England, 12.39–12.41, 12.43. Mr. K. Markham, Langport, England, 1.3, 1.20, 2.39, 3.13, 4.93, 7.39, 12.20. Dr. Craig McConnel, Colorado State University, Fort Collins, Colorado, USA, 4.83, 4.85. Dr. M. McLellan, University of Queensland, Australia, 9.5, 12.44, 12.47. Dr. C.A. Mebus, APHIS Plum Island Animal Disease Center, USA, 12.28. Dr. M. Miller, University of Missouri-Columbia, USA, 1.25, 4.98, 4.100, 5.19. Dr. A. Morrow, CTVM, Edinburgh, Scotland, 3.42, 3.43, 3.49, 12.33. Dr. C. Mortellaro, University of Milan, Italy, 7.59. Prof. M.T. Nassef, Assiut University, Egypt, 3.45. Dr. D.R. Nawathe, University of Maiduguri, Nigeria, 12.9. Dr. S. Nelson, University of Missouri-Columbia, USA, 2.23. Dr. P.S. Niehaus, Jerome, Idaho, USA, 7.113. Dr. J.K. O'Brien, University of Bristol, England, 3.67, 4.14, 7.76, 8.10, 9.22. Dr. G. Odiawo, University of Zimbabwe, Zimbabwe, 12.54–12.56. †Dr. O.E. Olsen, South Dakota State University, USA, 13.20. Mr. Peter Orpin, Leicester, England, 4.68. †Dr. Peter Ossent, University of Zürich, Switzerland, 7.13. Prof. A.L. Parodi, École Nationale Vétérinaire d'Alfort, France, 7.161, 7.162. †Prof. H. Pearson, University of Bristol, England, 1.10, 1.13, 4.77, 4.86, 6.4, 10.9, 10.22–10.24, 10.80, 12.75. Dr. Lyall Petrie, Western College of Veterinary Medicine, Saskatoon, Canada, 2.44, 3.28, 4.13, 4.61, 10.12, 10.13. †Mr. P.J.N. Pinsent, University of Bristol, England, 2.26, 2.46, 4.73, 7.102, 13.3. *Mr. G.C. Pritchard, VLA, Bury St Edmunds, England, 10.91*. Prof. G.H. Rautenbach, MEDUNSA, South Africa, 13.25. Dr. C.S. Ribble, Dept. of Population Medicine, University of Guelph, Guelph, Ontario, Canada, 1.9. Dr. A. Richardson, Harrogate, England, 1.6. Dr. J.M. Rutter, CVL, Weybridge, England, 5.10. Dr. D.W. Scott, New York State College of Veterinary Medicine, USA, 3.15, 3.18. †Dr. G.R. Scott, CTVM, Edinburgh, Scotland, 12.23, 12.25, 12.29. Dr. P.R. Scott, University of Edinburgh, Scotland, 9.2. Mr. A. Shakespeare, Dept. of Entomology and Dept. of Helminthology, Onderstepoort, VRI, South Africa, 3.31–3.33, 4.95, 4.96. Dr. M. Shearn, Institute for Animal Health, Compton, England, 11.32, 11.34, 11.38, 11.42. Dr. J.L. Shupe, Utah State University, USA, 13.21, 13.31, 13.32. Dr. Marian Smart, Western College of Veterinary Medicine, Saskatoon, Canada, 7.173. Mr. B.L. Smith, MAFTech Ruakura Agricultural Centre, New Zealand, 13.22, 13.23. Mr. S.E.G. Smith, Hoechst UK Ltd, Milton Keynes, England, 2.14, 9.44. Mr. J.B. Sproat, Castle Douglas, Scotland, 1.5, 1.7, 3.16, 3.69, 4.17, 4.36, 7.88, 8.25, 9.14, 9.37, 10.16, 10.29, 11.23, 12.66, 12.71, 12.79. †Mr. T.K. Stephens, Frome, England, 1.8, 2.48, 3.5, 3.11, 3.12, 4.4, 4.18, 4.87, 5.32, 7.12, 7.40, 7.45, 7.37, 7.91, 8.6, 8.18, 8.23, 10.54, 10.89, 11.5, 11.9, 11.31, 11.45. Heather Stevenson, SAC, Dumfries, Scotland, 12.71. Prof. M. Stöber, Clinic for Diseases of Cattle, Tierärztliche Hochschule Hannover, Germany, 9.27, 9.34. Mr. Ben Strugnell, VLA Thirsk, Yorkshire, 12.73*. Dr. S.M. Taylor, Veterinary Research Laboratories, Belfast, N. Ireland, 4.21, 4.94. Prof. H.M. Terblanche, MEDUNSA, South Africa, 10.26, 10.79. Dr. E. Teuscher, Lausanne, Switzerland, 12.57–12.60. Mr. I. Thomas, Llandeilo, Wales, 9.31. †Dr. E. Toussaint Raven, State University of Utrecht, Netherlands, 7.60. Mr. N. Twiddy, MAFF VI Centre, Lincoln, England, 7.154, 9.3, 9.39*. Dr. C.B. Usher, MSD Research Laboratories, São Paulo, Brazil, 3.53, 3.55. Veterinary Medical Diagnostic Laboratory, University of Missouri-Columbia, USA, 10.52, 12.18. Dr. W.M. Wass, Iowa State University, USA, 1.33, 1.34. †Mr. C.A. Watson, MAFF VI Centre, Bristol, England, 1.32*. Mr. C.L. Watson, Gloucester, England, 12.1, 12.8. Dr. D.G. White, Royal Veterinary College, England, 1.21, 3.44, 6.7, 7.95, 7.96, 12.42, 12.78. Dr. R. Whitlock, University of Pennsylvania, USA, 1.2, 1.24, 3.48, 4.29, 4.30, 4.60, 4.64, 4.71, 4.101, 7.72, 7.81, 7.94, 7.99, 7.114, 7.124, 7.126, 7.130, 7.159, 9.40, 12.69, 12.70, 12.81. Dr. Thomas Wittek, Veterinary Faculty, University of Glasgow, Scotland, 4.80, 4.81. Dr. W.A. Wolff, University of Missouri-Columbia, USA, 5.30, 5.35, 11.56. Dr. Kazunomi Yoshitani, Nanbu Livestock Hygiene Center, Hokkaido, Japan, 1.12.

Numerous illustrations have been published previously by Old Pond Publishing, Ipswich and CABI in *A Veterinary Book for Dairy Farmers*; Cattle Lameness and Hoofcare and Mastitis Control in Dairy Herds; 1.28, 9.7, 10.22, 10.24 and others by the *Veterinary Record* and *In Practice*; 8.14 and 9.29 by the *Canadian Veterinary Journal*; 13.27 and 13.28 by Stikstof, Netherlands; 10.32 by Iowa State Press; 11.24 by W B Saunders; and 10.22 and 10.23 by Baillière Tindall in *Veterinary Reproduction and Obstetrics*.

Again, gratitude is due to many clinical and pathological colleagues for useful advice and their readiness to be slide-quizzed; Christina McLachlan, Glasgow, is thanked for a mountain of secretarial help. Norma Blowey showed endless patience, food, and coffee during the joint revision sessions in Gloucester. Considerable help with the text has been given by Mr. Martyn Edelsten, Mr. Andy Holliman, Prof. Sheila Crispin and Dr. Nicola Gollnick, as well as Mr. Chris Livesey, Malton, Yorkshire, and Dr. Sian Mitchell, while Mr. P. Wragg of VLA Thirsk revised the microbiological nomenclature. Dr. Simon Bouisset, Dr. Enrico Chiavassa and Mr. John Sproat were particularly helpful with their provision of slides and comments on sections of the text.

Congenital disorders

Introduction

Congenital defects or diseases are abnormalities of structure or function that are present at birth. Not all congenital defects are caused by genetic factors. Some are due to environmental agents acting as teratogens. Examples include toxic plants (e.g., *Lupinus* species in crooked calf disease), prenatal viral infections (e.g., bovine virus diarrhea (BVD) resulting in cerebellar hypoplasia and hydrocephalus), and mineral deficiencies in dams of affected calves (e.g., manganese causing skeletal abnormalities).

Hereditary bovine defects are pathologically determined by mutant genes or chromosomal aberrations. Genetic defects are classified as lethal, sublethal, and subvital (including compatibility with life). Although typically occurring once or twice in every 500 births, a massive range of congenital disorders affecting different body systems has been identified in cattle, primarily as a result of records kept by artificial insemination (AI) organizations and breed societies. Economic losses are low overall, but abnormalities may cause considerable financial loss to individual pedigree breeders. Most congenital abnormalities are evident on external examination. About half of all calves with congenital defects are stillborn. Many of these stillbirths have no clearly established cause.

Examples of congenital defects are given by affected system. Some are single skeletal defects, others are systemic skeletal disorders such as chondrodysplasia. Certain congenital central nervous system (CNS) disorders may not manifest their first clinical effects until weeks or months after birth, e.g., spastic paresis and strabismus, respectively.

If several neonatal calves have similar defects, an epidemiological investigation is warranted. This should include the history of the dams (their nutrition and diseases, any drug therapy during gestation, and any movement of the dams onto premises with possible teratogens), and any possible relationship of season, newly introduced stock, as well as pedigree analysis.

Congenital ocular defects are considered elsewhere (Chapter 8), as are umbilical hernia (2.9), cryptorchidism (10.18), pseudohermaphroditism (10.40–10.42), and cerebellar hypoplasia (4.1, 4.2).

Cleft lip ("harelip", cheilognathoschisis); cleft palate (palatoschisis)

Definition: a failure of midline fusion during fetal development can lead to defects that affect different parts of the skeleton.

Clinical features: two obvious cranial abnormalities are illustrated here. A cleft lip in a young Shorthorn calf is shown in 1.1, in which a deep groove extends obliquely across the upper lip, nasolabial plate and jaw, involving not only skin but also bone (maxilla). This calf had

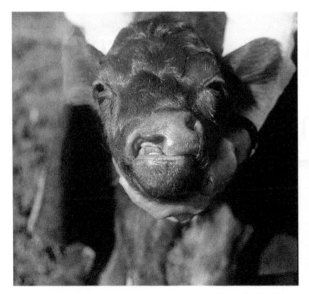

1.1. Cleft lip (Shorthorn calf) (USA)

extreme difficulty in sucking milk from the dam without considerable loss through regurgitation.

Cleft palate is seen as a congenital fissure of varying width in both the hard and soft palates of neonatal calves (1.2). The nasal turbinates (A) can be clearly seen through the fissure. The major presenting sign is nasal regurgitation, as seen in the Friesian calf (1.3). An aspiration pneumonia often develops early in life from inhalation of milk, sometimes while still nursing. Some calves with smaller fissures may appear clinically normal during suckling because the teat when in the calf's mouth, closes the fissure. Clinical signs are seen when it starts to eat solid food. Cleft palate is often associated with other congenital defects, particularly arthrogryposis (1.15). The Holstein calf (1.2) was a "bulldog" (see 1.6). Other midline defects include spina bifida (1.20) and ventricular septal defect (1.30, 1.31).

Meningocele

The large, red, fluid-filled sac (1.4) is the meninges protruding through a midline cleft in the frontal bones. The sac contains cerebrospinal fluid. The calf, a 4-day-old Hereford crossbred bull, was otherwise healthy. An inherited defect was unlikely in this case (see also 1.20).

Salivary mucocele

Definition: extravasation of saliva into subcutaneous tissues.

Clinical features: this Limousin x Friesian heifer (1.5) had shown this soft, painless, fluctuating swelling since birth. In other cases it develops in the first few weeks of life.

Differential diagnosis: calf diphtheria (2.42), submandibular abscess (4.51).

1.2. Cleft palate (Holstein calf) (USA)

Achondroplastic dwarfism ("bulldog calf") or dyschondroplasia

Definition: a failure of cartilaginous growth usually as an inherited defect.

Clinical features: the Hereford calf (1.6) demonstrates brachycephalic dwarfism. The head is short and abnormally broad, the lower jaw is overshot, and the legs are very short. The abdomen was also enlarged. The calf had difficulty in standing, was dyspneic as a result of the skull deformity ("snorter dwarf"), and a cleft palate was also present. A 2-week-old Simmental crossbred suckler calf (1.7) shows severe bowing of all four legs, especially forelegs, stunting, and a slightly dished face, and euthanasia was indicated. Born in May from a winter-housed dam fed only silage, extra feed appeared to reduce the incidence of achondroplasia from 40/200 to 5/200 offspring in successive years.

Bulldog calves are often born dead (1.8). This Ayrshire has a large head and short legs, but also has extensive subcutaneous edema (anasarca). Dwarfism is inherited in several breeds, including Hereford and Angus.

A related condition is congenital joint laxity and dwarfism (CJLD), which is a distinct congenital anomaly in Canada and the UK. A severe CJLD case from Canada,

1.3. Cleft palate with nasal regurgitation (Friesian calf)

1.5. Salivary mucocele (Limousin x Friesian)

the newborn calf (1.9) has a crouched appearance, short legs, metacarpophalangeal hyperextension, and sickle-shaped hind legs. Many calves are disproportionate dwarfs. The joints become stable within 2 weeks and the calves can then walk normally. Other abnormalities are not seen. In the UK in 2009/10, 70 of a group of 85 South Devon x Angus calves showed shortened limbs, joint laxity (especially of the fetlocks), dyspnea in the first days

1.4. Meningocele (Hereford cross, 4 days old)

1.6. Brachycephalic dwarfism (Hereford)

1.7. Brachycephalic dwarfism (Simmental cross)

1.8. Brachycephalic dwarfism "bulldog calf" (Ayrshire)

of life, and in a few cases brachygnathia. The dams had been fed straw after housing, and later straw and silage.

Schistosomus reflexus

One calf of twins was a normal live calf and the other was a schistosomus reflexus (1.10). The hindquarters are twisted towards the head, the ventral abdominal wall is open, and the viscera are exposed. This anomaly usually causes dystocia, often requiring correction by cesarian section.

1.9. Congenital joint laxity and dwarfism (Hereford) (Canada)

1.10. Schistosomus reflexus and normal twin (Hereford cross)

Hydranencephaly

The cerebral hemispheres are absent and their site is occupied by cerebrospinal fluid. The fluid has been drained from this specimen (1.11) after removal of the meninges. Hydranencephaly and arthrogryposis occur as a combined defect in epidemic form following certain intrauterine viral infections, e.g., Akabane virus (1.12)

1.11. Hydranencephaly showing exposed brain (Japan)

1.12. Hydranencephaly and arthrogryposis in Akabane virus (Japan)

1.14. Contracted foreleg flexor tendons (Hereford cross)

Schmallenberg virus (12.82). This calf with both arthrogryposis and hydranencephaly died shortly after birth.

Hydrocephalus

The cranium (1.13) is enlarged due to pressure from an excessive volume of cerebrospinal fluid within the ventricular system. Though usually congenital in calves, it also can occur as a rare acquired condition in adult cattle, through infection or trauma. In one form of bovine hydrocephalus there is achondroplastic dishing of the face and a foreshortened maxilla ("bulldog", see 1.6).

Contracted tendons

Considered as the most prevalent musculoskeletal abnormality of neonatal calves, congenital contraction of the flexor tendons in this neonatal Hereford crossbred calf (1.14) has caused excessive flexion of the carpal and fetlock joints in the forelimbs. The hind legs are placed under the body to improve weightbearing. The affected joints may be manually extended. Pectoral amyotonia is frequently present. Some forms of the condition are inherited through an autosomal recessive gene. Rarely, cases are associated with cleft palate (1.2).

Management: mild cases recover without treatment, although affected calves should be regularly lifted into the standing position as a form of physiotherapy. Moderate cases can be splinted, and severely affected calves may need surgery (tenotomy of one or both flexors). The prognosis is poor if marked carpal flexion is present.

Arthrogryposis

Arthrogryposis (1.15) is an extreme form of contracted tendons, in which many joints are fixed in flexion or extension (ankylosed). Frequently, two, three, or all four limbs are involved in various combinations of flexion and extension. This calf has torticollis. The left foreleg is rotated about 180° (note the position of the dewclaws) and the right hind leg is sickle-shaped. Many such fetuses cause dystocia if carried to term. Some cases involve an *in utero* viral infection, e.g., BVD (p. 54), Akabane virus (p. 4), or they may be associated with the CVM (complex vertebral malformation) gene.

Complex vertebral malformation (CVM)

A lethal genetic defect in a single recessive gene that in most cases causes fetal resorption, abortion, or stillbirths, and hence affected cattle, usually Holsteins, have reduced

1.13. Hydrocephalus (Hereford cross)

1.15. Arthrogryposis and torticollis (Friesian)

1

1.16. CVM cow

1.18. Atresia ani

fertility, manifesting as poor conception rates. Surviving animals may show skeletal malformations such as a foreshortened neck and thorax, deformed carpal and metacarpal joints, and, as in 1.16, a distortion, twisting, and hypoplasia of the tail. The defective gene has now largely been bred out.

Vertebral fusion and kyphosis

Fusion of most of the cervical, thoracic, and lumbar vertebrae in this 2-week-old Holstein calf (1.17) was associated with a shortened neck and increased convex curvature of the spine (kyphosis). The etiology is unknown. Kyphosis may be an inherited or acquired condition (see 7.94). It is often not apparent at birth, but progressively deteriorates with age. Mild cases will reach slaughter weight. Severe cases are best culled.

Atresia ani

Congenital absence of the anus (1.18) is manifested clinically by an absence of feces, and the gradual development of abdominal distension. A small dimple may indicate the position of the anal sphincter. If the rectum is present, some calves may have a soft bulge from the pressure of accumulating feces and these may be treated

surgically. Calves usually show marked colic within 3 days. A fistula sometimes develops between the rectum and urogenital tract (see also 2.15).

Hypoplastic tail ("wry tail")

One of the more common congenital conditions. This calf (1.19) was born with no tail and with part of the coccyx absent. It could walk normally and reached slaughter weight. Other animals with more severe coccygeal hypoplasia develop an unsteady rolling gait that becomes progressively more severe with age, and are hence best culled.

Spina bifida

Definition: defect of the two halves of the vertebral arch, through which the spinal cord and meninges may or may not protrude.

Clinical features: severe posterior paresis is seen in this Friesian neonate (1.20). The red, raised, and circumscribed protuberance in the sacral region involves a myelomeningocele (protrusion of both cord and meninges). The congenital defect is due to an absence of the dorsal portion of the spine (compare 1.4). Even if ataxia is not

1.17. Vertebral fusion and kyphosis (Holstein, 2 weeks old) (Belgium)

1.19. Hypoplastic tail

1.20. Spina bifida with paresis (Friesian calf)

1.22. Segmental jejunal aplasia and stenosis (Charbray)

severe, affected calves are best culled due to the risk of ascending spinal infection.

Hypospadia

In this rare, male, congenital developmental anomaly, the urethra opens onto the perineum below the anus (1.21). The rudimentary penis is seen as a pink groove. There is urine staining of the inguinal region below.

Segmental jejunal aplasia, atresia coli

To the right, the proximal jejunum (A) is grossly distended with fluid, as the calf (1.22), a 1-week-old Charbray, initially suckled normally. The distal jejunum (B) is empty owing to jejunal aplasia and stenosis. Meconium was present in the large intestine. The calf had developed progressive abdominal distension from 4 days old. A typical clinical sign is the passage of small amounts of rectal mucus, as shown in 1.23, where both of these 3-day-old Charolais cross twins were affected.

Other cases of intestinal aplasia can involve the ileum, colon, and rectum, producing similar signs. Atresia coli calves appear normal at birth, rapidly develop abdominal distension and die within 1 week, with the small intestine and cecum grossly distended and the colon empty. However, proximal intestinal obstruction tends to produce a more acute and rapidly progressive condition. In some cases the intestine opens into the abdominal cavity, causing peritonitis and death within 48 hours.

Differential diagnosis: Intussusception jejunal (4.86), jejunal torsion and intussusception (4.87), perforated abomasal ulcer (2.28), gut stasis from enterotoxemia.

Syndactyly ("mule foot")

The claws of both forelegs of this Holstein bull calf (1.24) are fused. This congenital defect is due to homozygosity of a simple autosomal recessive gene with incomplete penetrance. It is the most common inherited skeletal defect of US Holstein cattle, but also occurs in several other breeds. One or more limbs may be affected.

Epitheliogenesis imperfecta

A congenital absence of skin, in this case (1.25) involving the digital horn, seen most clearly in the hind feet. In a young Holstein calf (1.26), the extensive loss of digital

1.21. Hypospadia (Friesian bull calf)

1.23. Anal mucus from intestinal obstruction

1.24.   Syndactyly ("mule foot") (Holstein, USA)

1.26.   Epitheliogenesis imperfecta (Holstein)

horn, which involved all four limbs, is obvious. It is a rare sublethal defect in various breeds, inherited as a simple autosomal recessive gene. Large epithelial defects can affect the distal parts of the limbs as well as the muzzle, tongue and hard palate. Bleeding and secondary infection can lead to septicemia and early death.

Hypotrichosis

In one form of this inherited condition, viable hypotrichosis, the coat hair is thin, wavy and silky (1.27). The wrinkled skin (A) is only 2–3 cells thick. The calf has several areas of abraded skin including the carpus and the elbow. A simple autosomal recessive trait is recorded in

1.25.   Epitheliogenesis imperfecta digital horn (Angus) (USA)

1.27.   Hypotrichosis (Simmental cross, USA)

1.28. Parakeratosis (Friesian cross, 5 weeks old)

1.29. Baldy calf syndrome (Hereford cross)

Herefords. In another form, lethal hypotrichosis, calves, usually hairless, are born dead or die shortly afterwards.

Parakeratosis (adema disease, lethal trait A46)

An inherited defect, which in Friesian-type cattle is associated with a poor intestinal uptake of zinc. Calves develop conjunctivitis, diarrhea, and an increased susceptibility to infection, and eventually die unless treated. This calf (1.28), normal at birth, developed a generalized parakeratosis at 5 weeks old. The skin of the head and neck has become thickened with scales, cracks, and fissures. Above the eye, the underlying surface is raw and abraded.

Differential diagnosis: dermatophilosis (3.37–3.43), severe lice infestation (pediculosis) (3.20–3.24). Diagnosis confirmed by response to zinc therapy.

Management: calves should be culled (lethal trait).

Baldy calf syndrome

A congenital disorder that is mainly seen in Holsteins, baldy calf syndrome is associated with hypotrichosis. The autosomal recessive trait is lethal in male Holsteins, while heifers show signs within a few weeks. This Hereford-cross calf (1.29) was severely depressed, with pyrexia, poor appetite, lacrimation, and nasal discharge. Areas of alopecia appeared over the head and neck. Most cases are destroyed owing to chronic unthriftiness. Both baldy calf syndrome and parakeratosis (1.28) respond to oral zinc supplementation, but relapse when this is stopped.

Ventricular septal defect (VSD)

This 2-day-old Friesian calf had a VSD (1.30). It was lethargic and dyspneic, especially on exercise, had

pronounced tachycardia, and showed hyperemia of the muzzle. It died 2 days later. Small defects may produce few clinical effects except a loud systolic murmur. Affected calves commonly have difficulty drinking their milk, and may develop severe dyspnea and/or rumen bloat from esophageal groove failure.

In a severe case revealed at autopsy, note the patency of the ventricular septum (1.31). The position of the left

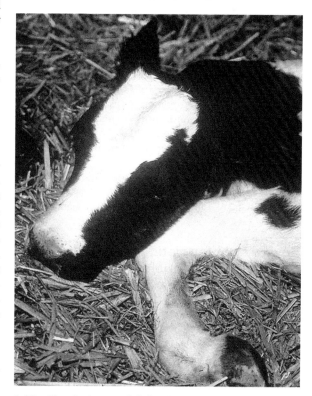

1.30. Ventricular septal defect (Friesian, 2 days old)

1.31. Ventricular septal defect

1.32. Patent ductus arteriosus (Charolais bull calf, 18 days old)

atrioventricular (AV) valves (A) shows that the opening involves the membranous portion of the septum. Blood is usually shunted left to right. VSD may be combined with other cardiovascular anomalies.

Patent ductus arteriosus (PDA)

The heart of a crossbred Charolais bull calf (1.32), which suddenly collapsed with signs of severe tachypnea when 18 days old, shows an opening (A) (internal diameter 2.5 mm) between the aortic trunk (B) and the pulmonary artery (C). Scissors point to the PDA. Forceps have been placed between the left ventricle (bottom) and the aorta to show normal blood flow.

This opening usually closes soon after birth. If it remains patent, unoxygenated blood can pass from the pulmonary trunk into the aorta, producing signs similar to a VSD.

Bovine erythropoietic porphyria, congenital erythropoietic porphyria (BEP, CEP, "pink tooth")

Definition: genetic condition, simple autosomal recessive, with an accumulation of porphyrin-type isomers, resulting in photosensitization developing in various breeds (e.g., Holstein, Shorthorn, Ayrshire, Hereford).

Clinical features: more common than BEPP (see below) and resulting in more severe photosensitization,

other signs include red-brown discoloration of teeth (1.33), bones (ribs, 1.34), and urine (which have a high concentration of uroporphyrins). Teeth and urine fluoresce under Woods lamp. A regenerative anemia and stunted growth are also seen.

Differential diagnosis: other forms of photosensitization including BEPP (where red-brown teeth are not evident). See also pp. 30, 253, 254.

Management: breeding policy, namely elimination of affected carriers, and indoor confinement of affected stock for beef.

1.33. Erythropoietic porphyria (BEP) (USA)

1.34. Erythropoietic porphyria: fluorescence in ribs (USA)

1.36. Amorphous globosus

Bovine erythropoietic protoporphyria (BEPP)

Definition: sporadic genetic condition (possibly auto-somal recessive) causing photosensitization as a result of ferrochelatase deficiency causing raised levels of proto-porphyrins in red cells and body tissues. Protoporphyrin

1.35. Erythropoietic protoporphyria (BEPP): muzzle and tongue changes

is a photodynamic agent. Reported in Limousin and Blonde d'Aquitaine breeds.

Clinical features: major signs are photodermatitis and photophobia with the severity being greater in younger cattle. A 2-week-old Limousin crossbred suckler calf (1.35) shows marked erythema, ulceration and scabs on the nares and ear tips, sublingual ulceration and drooling as a result of oral discomfort.

Differential diagnosis: other forms of photosensitization (see p. 30, 253).

Management: breeding policy should avoid and cull known carriers. Affected calves should be reared indoors to avoid sunlight.

Amorphous globosus

This extreme form of congenital abnormality (1.36), which is normally born twin to a healthy calf, consisted of a skin covering and internally a rudimentary heart and lungs. The navel cord is clearly seen at the base.

Neonatal disorders

Introduction

This chapter covers disorders of the calf from birth until postweaning. The first section deals with navel ill, umbilical hernia, and general conditions of the navel. Later sections cover different forms of diarrhea and alopecia, with a miscellaneous group including calf diphtheria and joint ill. According to the presenting signs, other diseases of calfhood are considered in the relevant chapters; for example, lice, ringworm, and skin diseases are to be found in Chapter 3, respiratory problems in Chapter 5, and meningitis in Chapter 9.

A calf mortality rate of 5% of live births is considered to be an acceptable figure. A "target" neonatal mortality rate could be 3%. Much higher losses may occur where husbandry and management are poor. There are many reasons why the young calf is particularly susceptible to disease. Its immunological defense mechanisms are not fully developed. It will be going through the transition from passive to active immunity. The abomasum is less acidic, especially in the first few days of life, and this reduces the rate of kill of enterobacteriaciae and other ingested organisms. The calf may have several changes of diet. Moreover, the navel provides an additional early route by which infection may enter the body. Many calf diseases are exacerbated by failure to provide adequate housing, management, or colostral intake.

Conditions of umbilicus (navel)

Umbilical eventration

Clinical features: umbilical eventration is seen in a small proportion of calves immediately after birth. The prolapsed intestines (jejunum) may be fully exposed, as in the Friesian (2.1), or contained in a sac of peritoneum. Opening the sac in a Charolais calf revealed a congested intestine (2.2). Often the exposed intestine ruptures when the calf moves. The prognosis is then hopeless. In more advanced and exposed cases the intestinal loops turn a deep red/purple color due to ischemic necrosis (2.1).

Management: except in the very recent (<3 hours) case, surgery is rarely warranted.

Navel ill (omphalophlebitis)

Definition: inflammation, usually by infection, of the tissues of the umbilicus.

Clinical features: lacking skin or any other protective layer, the moist, fleshy navel cord is particularly prone to infection until it dries up, normally within 1 week of birth. In the first calf (2.3) (shown at 3 days old) the enlarged and still moist navel cord is seen entering an

2.1. Umbilical eventration with jejunum (Friesian)

2.3. Navel ill (omphalophlebitis) (Friesian, 3 days old)

inflamed and swollen umbilical ring. Navel ill is uncommon at this age.

The more typical case is pyrexic, with a swollen, painful navel exuding a foul-smelling creamy-white pus (2.4). Culture usually reveals a mixed bacterial flora including *Escherichia coli*, *Proteus*, *Staphylococcus*, and *Arcanobacterium pyogenes*. This case persisted for several weeks.

Alopecia on the medial aspects of the thighs (2.5) is due to a combination of urine scald and excessive cleansing of the navel by the owner. Some cases show no gross discharge, but the tip of the swollen navel will be moist and malodorous.

In other cases an intra-abdominal abscess may develop in the omphalic (umbilical) vein. In 2.6, A shows the intra-abdominal abscess in the grossly distended umbilical vein, adjacent to the navel, B. Spontaneous rupture of the abscess can lead to death from peritonitis, as in this calf. Occasional cases involve the urachus to produce a cystitis which can lead to stunted growth, sickness, and death several months after birth.

Septicemia can result in localization of infection in the joints (2.48, 2.49), meninges, endocardium, or end-arteries of limbs.

Differential diagnosis: umbilical hernia (2.9), eventration (2.1), granuloma (2.7).

Management: cleansing, removal of necrotic tissue, drainage, including use of a catheter to perform deep flushing of intra-abdominal lesions, and prolonged

2.2. Umbilical eventration with jejunum (Charolais)

2.4. Navel ill with purulent exudate

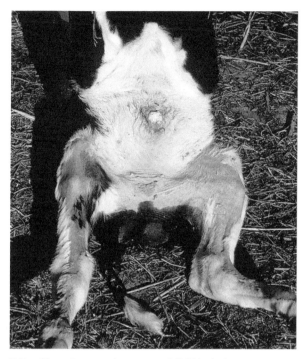

2.5. Alopecia secondary to navel ill (Friesian)

systemic antibiotics. Prevention involves improved hygiene at calving, routine use of topical dressings to disinfect and desiccate the moist navel cord, and optimal colostral intake.

Umbilical granuloma

Definition: a tumor-like mass of granulation tissue due to a chronic inflammatory process at the navel.

Clinical features: a small bifurcated mass of granulation tissue protrudes from the navel of this 2-week-old calf (2.7). Many cases consist of a single mass of tissue. It is only slightly painful and affected calves are generally not pyrexic, although there may be superficial infection present, as in this case. The condition will not resolve

2.6. Autopsy with omphalic venous abscessation and peritonitis

2.7. Umbilical granuloma (Hereford cross)

2.8. Large umbilical granuloma

until the mass is removed by ligation at its base. If left untreated (2.8), it will persist into adult life.

Umbilical hernia

Clinical features: a large, soft, and fluctuating ventral abdominal swelling can be seen in this 3-month-old Friesian calf (2.9). The arched back in this calf clearly

2.9. Umbilical hernia

2

2.10. Jejunal loops in strangulated umbilical hernia

2.12. Umbilical abscess and rumen fistula (Friesian, 3 months old)

depicts discomfort. Many smaller hernias are not associated with pain. Rarely, in moderate-sized umbilical hernias, the jejunal loops become strangulated, and the calf is in severe pain, becomes toxemic, and dies within a day or two. Autopsy of one such case (2.10) shows the multiple loops with severe serosal hemorrhage. Although present from birth, some hernias are not noticed until the calf is at least 2–3 weeks old. A proportion of cases are inherited. Irreducible and strangulated hernias are uncommon.

Differential diagnosis: navel abscess (2.11), urolithiasis (10.7), ruptured urethra (10.7).

Management: small hernial rings often close within 6 months and do not require treatment. Large hernias require corrective surgery.

Umbilical abscess

Clinical features: the swelling in this 4-month-old Friesian male (2.11) is cranial to the prepuce (compare urolithiasis (10.7), where it is caudal), and appeared

spontaneously. The mass was initially hard, hot, and painful. Pyrexia led to systemic illness. Parenteral antibiotics resulted in a change to a more fluctuating swelling, which was successfully lanced and drained.

A hernia and an umbilical abscess can occur together. Occasionally, navel ill or navel abscess produces a localized peritonitis that erodes through the rumen wall to produce a rumenal fistula. 2.12 shows a 3-month-old Friesian male with a grossly enlarged navel sac, soiled anteriorly. Rumen contents leaked through the fistula, shown in close-up in 2.13.

Differential diagnosis: navel ill (2.3), umbilical hernia (2.9), rectourethral fistula (2.15).

Management: careful investigation is needed to define any intra-abdominal involvement such as a urachal abscess. Exploratory surgery, with guarded prognosis.

Navel suckling

Navel suckling (2.14) is a common vice in group-housed, bucket-fed calves, especially if they are in poor condition

2.11. Umbilical abscess (Friesian, 4 months old)

2.13. Enlarged view of umbilical rumen fistula

2.14. Navel suckling

and have intercurrent diseases. The calf being sucked has an enlarged navel, which could be infected. There is hair loss around the navel, indicating a chronic problem. The ears, tail, and scrotum can also be suckled.

Management: rear calves in single pens until 1 week postweaning. Feed milk from teats, not bucket. Control intercurrent disease.

Rectourethral umbilical fistula

Note the very soiled hair around the navel and prepuce, and the discolored urine in this 2-day-old Holstein male (2.15).

Differential diagnosis: this rare condition may be confused with navel ill and pervious urachus.

Management: spontaneous resolution does not occur. Surgical correction is usually impossible.

2.15. Rectourethral fistula (Holstein, 2 days old)

Conditions of gastrointestinal tract

Calf scour

Etiology and pathogenesis: enteritis and diarrhea in calves are major causes of death in the first few weeks of life. A wide range of agents can be involved, some producing diarrhea with or without dehydration, others leading to systemic involvement. Diarrhea in the first few days of life is commonly caused by bacterial infections, for example, *E. coli* or *Clostridium perfringens*. Their toxins lead to hypersecretion from the intestine and subsequent fluid loss, seen as diarrhea. Viral infections (rotavirus and coronavirus) and *Cryptosporidia* typically occur at 10–14 days (as maternal colostral antibody wanes), and are considered the major causes of calf scour. Diarrhea occurs because the intestinal wall is damaged, preventing resorption of fluid. *Salmonella* scouring can occur at any age.

The role of other agents (e.g., parvovirus, Breda virus, a calici-like virus, and astrovirus, BVD, and IBR viruses) in the calf scour syndrome has not been well defined.

Management: hygiene, colostrum, and good feeding practices are very important for control. Vaccines are available against *E. coli*, rotavirus, coronavirus, and *Salmonella*. It is not possible to differentiate fully between the various causes of scour on the basis of gross appearance and clinical signs alone, although the following illustrations give a few guidelines.

Rotavirus, coronavirus, and *Cryptosporidia*

Clinical features: the majority of calves become infected with rotavirus, coronavirus, and *Cryptosporidia*, but normally only those subjected to a heavy challenge or concurrent disease show clinical signs. The cross-bred Limousin calf (2.16) is bright and alert, but has pasty yellow diarrhea around the tail. Both rotavirus and *Cryptosporidia* were identified in the feces. Increased mucus may be passed. There may be tenesmus with *Cryptosporidia*. More advanced cases (2.17) show dehydration and general systemic involvement such as sunken eyes, a dry muzzle, hyperemia of the nares, and a purulent nasal discharge. At autopsy 2 days later, the colon was thickened, corrugated, and exuding blood (2.18). *Cryptosporidia*, rotavirus, coronavirus, and enterotoxigenic *E. coli* (responsible for the hemorrhagic colitis) were all isolated.

White scour

Clinical features: "white scour" occurs when intestinal damage is such that partially digested white milk is passed in the feces. Note the characteristic white fecal soiling of the flanks and tail in this 3-week-old Holstein heifer (2.19). Originally considered to be part

2

2.16. Calf scour with rotavirus and cryptosporidial infection (Limousin cross)

2.19. White scour (Holstein, 3 weeks old)

2.17. Severe calf scour with rotavirus, coronavirus, and *E. coli* (USA)

of the colibacillosis syndrome, it is now known that white scour can result from various agents, including rotavirus. Voluminous, white, rotavirus-positive feces can be voided during an explosive outbreak in a calf unit (2.20).

Enterotoxemia

Clinical features: *Clostridium perfringens* enterotoxemia normally affects calves in the first few days of life. The small intestine (A) on the left of 2.21 shows a dark-red ischemic necrosis. Other areas (B) are gas-filled, which is indicative of gut stasis and gas formation. Following sudden death, type C enterotoxin was demonstrated.

2.18. Autopsy of calf in 2.17 with thickened hemorrhagic colon (USA)

2.20. Feces in explosive outbreak of white scour

2.21. *C. perfringens* enterotoxemia at autopsy (USA)

2.24. Feces with *S. enterica* serovar *Typhimurium* (Friesian, 3 weeks old)

Salmonellosis

Definition: a widespread contagious disease caused by *Salmonella* spp., localized in almost any organ, leading to enteritis, septicemia, arthritis, and meningitis. *S. enterica*, serovar *Typhimurium* is most common, but many other serovars may be involved.

Clinical features: a 1-week-old crossbred Hereford calf (2.22) is moribund and passing dysenteric feces, a mixture of blood, mucus, and intestinal mucosal lining. Classically, necropsy revealed a diphtheritic enteritis (2.23), with thickening of the mucosa. However, not all

calves are affected so severely. Although *Salmonella enterica*, serovar *Typhimurium* was isolated from the dysenteric feces of the affected 3-week-old Friesian calf (2.24), it was only mildly ill. Other cases show slight intestinal inflammation, the main changes being lung congestion and epicardial and renal hemorrhages. Animals recovering from peracute septicemia (especially *S. dublin*) may occasionally develop necrosis of the extremities, particularly in the ear tips, tail and legs. The 4-month-old Friesian (2.25) was recovering from a nonspecific pyrexia that had affected it some 6 weeks previously. Enteritis had not been observed, and is often not involved, but later ear tip necrosis produced a bilateral slough of more than half of the pinna. *S. dublin* was isolated from the feces. In the 4-month-old crossbred Hereford (2.26), circumferential skin necrosis immediately above the hind fetlocks has produced gangrene and necrosis of the extremities. Over-extension at the fetlocks is probably due to flexor tendon rupture. Salivation is a pain response.

2.22. Salmonellosis dysenteric feces (Hereford cross, 1 week old)

2.23. Autopsy of calf with salmonellosis showing diphtheritic enteritis (USA)

2.25. Necrosis of ear tips in peracute septicemia (Friesian)

2

2.26. Gangrene and skin necrosis of distal limb (Hereford cross, 4 months old)

2.27. Acute abomasitis (Friesian, 2 weeks old)

Differential diagnosis: many other causes of enteritis including digestive upsets, *E. coli* septicemia (p. 17), coccidiosis (2.32), ergot poisoning (7.159), constricting wire around leg (7.156).

Management: treatment should include fluids and electrolyte solutions given orally or in severe cases intravenously. Prophylaxis includes isolation of diseased calves, improved hygiene and adequate colostral intake in the first 6 hours after birth. Dam vaccination protects against enteritis, septicemia, and abortion, and also reduces *Salmonella* excretion rates in both dam and calf. Calves may also be vaccinated. Thorough cleansing and disinfection between batches, including "all in/all out" systems, as well as vermin control are important in eliminating reservoirs of *Salmonella*. The zoonotic risk should always be borne in mind.

Abomasal ulceration

Clinical features: in calves the majority of abomasal ulcers are subclinical, and may be associated with irregular feeding, overfeeding, and/or overconsumption of dry feed. More advanced cases show low-grade abdominal pain, developing into peritonitis if the ulcer perforates.

The 2-week-old Friesian (2.27) was moribund, with drooping ears, sunken eyes, and regurgitated rumen contents on its lips. It died within hours. Autopsy revealed an acute abomasitis with two perforated ulcers (2.28) with a creamy-white necrotic lining. Death was due to acute peritonitis (2.29). Fibrin and food coat the serosal surface of an inflamed and dilated small intestine. Abomasal ulcers are also seen in adult cattle (4.72, 4.73), in veal calves and in thriving beef calves, 2–4 months old, at pasture.

Differential diagnosis: includes salmonellosis (2.22), BVD, peritonitis, intestinal obstruction.

Management: metoclopramide has been given to control abomasal bloat. NSAIDs, anti-inflammatory

drugs, and antibiotics aid control of inflammation and ulceration.

Prevention: avoid overfeeding, sudden dietary changes, and excessive milk flow rates through teats.

Abomasal dilatation and torsion

Definition: atony of the abomasum is followed by gaseous distension, then by torsion. Both may be secondary to abomasal ulceration.

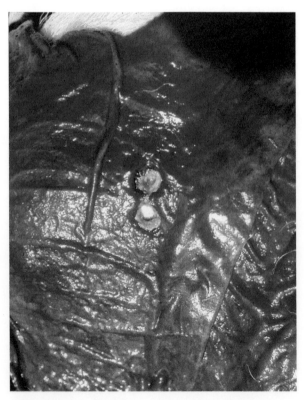

2.28. Autopsy of 2.27 with two perforating ulcers and acute abomasitis

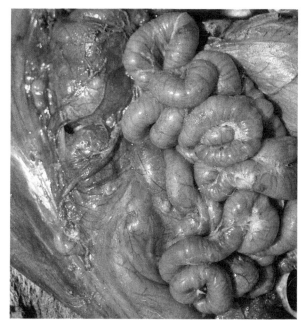

2.29. Acute peritonitis following abomasal perforation

Clinical signs: often sudden in onset. In the acute syndrome affected calves develop severe abomasal tympany, with loud splashing sounds audible from the excess fluid present. A surgical view of a typical distended abomasum filled with gas and fluid is seen in 2.30. Shock develops quickly, and affected calves are often found collapsed. Many cases, however, develop spontaneously even when single suckled.

Management: metoclopramide, NSAIDs, anti-inflammatory drugs, antibiotics, and nursing. Surgery (successful in 2.30) may be attempted on high-value animals.

Differential diagnosis: abomasal tympany is almost pathognomonic, ruminal tympany.

Prevention: avoid overfeeding and sudden dietary changes.

Other abdominal conditions
Coccidiosis

Definition: coccidiosis is an infection of the lower small intestine, cecum, colon, and rectum, caused by the protozoan parasite *Eimeria*. A wide range of species are involved, with *E. zuernii* and *E. bovis* being the most pathogenic. Infestations in the small intestine are considered to be less pathogenic due to the more rapid cellular regeneration than in the large intestine, and because the large intestine provides a further opportunity for the resorption of water.

Clinical features: disease is usually associated with calves crowded in damp and unhygienic conditions. Adult animals (e.g., suckler cows) may be carriers, though oocysts may survive many months in the environment. The incubation period is 17–21 days. Affected calves are dull, pyrexic, and typically produce watery feces, usually mixed with blood. Tenesmus (2.31), with continued straining and frequent passage of small quantities of blood and feces, is a characteristic sign. The anal sphincter is open, exposing the rectal mucosa. Hair loss on the inside of the leg results from fecal soiling. Another calf (2.32) shows a thickened and inflamed colonic mucosa. Blood on the surface of freshly passed feces unrelated to coccidiosis, is a normal feature of some calves, but it occurs more often following stress, e.g., transport, or sale through a livestock market.

Differential diagnosis: diagnosis depends on clinical signs, the demonstration of oocysts on fecal flotation or direct smear, and autopsy changes such as thickening and inflammation of the intestinal mucosa. Normal non-affected calves may excrete lower numbers of oocysts.

2.30. Abomasal torsion at celiotomy (Italy)

2.31. Coccidiosis with severe tenesmus and bloody feces

2.32. Coccidiosis showing thickened hemorrhagic colon (USA)

2.34. Crusty muzzle changes in necrotic enteritis (beef calf, 2 months old)

Differentials include salmonellosis (2.22–2.24), BVD (4.3), and necrotic enteritis (see below).

Management: treatment includes oral decoquinate, toltrazuril, amprolium or sulfaquinoxaline, and parenteral sulfonamides in advanced cases. Prevention is by management changes to avoid fecal contamination of feed, cleaning between batches using an ammonia-based disinfectant or other suitable oocide, and by strategic use of coccidiostats soon after the expected period of exposure.

Necrotic enteritis

Clinical features: this relatively recently recognized disease of 2–4-month-old suckled beef calves in the UK has an unknown etiology. Affected calves show intense dullness of demeanor (2.33), often with drooping ears, an arched back from abdominal pain, and a profuse black/brown scour. Other major signs are tenesmus with diarrhea or dysentery, and prominent nasal and oral lesions, which are grossly typical of mucosal disease but calves have no BVD antigen. Typical crusty muzzle

changes are seen in 2.34, while autopsy exposes the extent of pharyngeal and laryngeal necrosis (2.35). The serosal surfaces of the small intestine (2.36) show fibrin overlying extensive hemorrhagic areas. These changes extend into the muscular and mucosal layers. Other internal viscera also have hemorrhages (e.g., kidney, abomasum, lungs).

Differential diagnosis: coccidiosis (2.31), abomasal ulceration (2.28), salmonellosis (2.22). The autopsy findings are diagnostic (2.35, 2.36).

Management: supportive therapy with NSAIDs, fluid therapy, and antibiotics, but prognosis is poor.

Periweaning calf diarrhea syndrome

Definition: a chronic low-grade brown digestive scour in calves before or after weaning, commonly on a group basis.

2.33. Necrotic enteritis. Calf is dull with arched back and profuse scour

2.35. Autopsy showing pharyngeal and laryngeal necrosis in necrotic enteritis

2.36. Autopsy showing fibrin overlying hemorrhagic jejunum in necrotic enteritis

Clinical features: initially feces appear slightly loose. As the condition progresses, a brown "pastey" diarrhea is seen, with pronounced weight loss. Within group morbidity is high but mortality is low. On autopsy, the large intestine is grossly dilated and the contents watery. The 7-week-old white Friesian calf in the center of 2.37 is in poor condition, with its tail and perineum matted with feces. This is typical of the syndrome. These calves were fed unsuitable protein in a concentrate intended for adult cattle, and remained stunted for many months. Infection with *Giardia* and *Campylobacter* species has been implicated in some cases.

Differential diagnosis: digestive upsets, coccidiosis, enteric salmonellosis.

Management: improve rumen development by feeding well-balanced, high-quality rations. Inadequate intakes of concentrates preweaning may retard ruminal development. "Coarse mix" rations may produce fewer problems than pellets by reducing eating rate and increasing chewing and salivation. High-starch and low-fiber diets leading to rumen acidosis predispose to periweaning diarrhea, as will irregular feeding, poor rumen development, and antinutrient factors such as excessive levels of wheat gluten and trypsin inhibitors in soya. Improve hygiene. Badly affected

2.37. Perianal soiling in periweaning calf diarrhea

2.38. Severe ruminal tympany and periweaning calf diarrhea (Hereford cross, 7 weeks old)

calves should be returned to a whole milk diet. Treatment with antibacterial and antiprotozoal agents such as decoquinate toltrazuril and sulfonamides may be useful.

Ruminal tympany in calves

Definition: accumulation of gas in the rumen in the milk-fed calf, and an associated rumenal atony.

Clinical features: rumen bloat is most commonly seen 1–2 hours after feeding milk or milk substitute, and is often associated with a pasty scour and bouts of colic, sometimes quite severe. It commonly results from feeding errors that lead to incomplete esophageal groove closure. Milk entering the rumen ferments and produces bloat with severe colic. Most incidents have a high morbidity but low mortality. The 4-week-old Hereford cross calf (2.38) shows severe ruminal tympany, with soiling of the tail and perineum, associated with chronic diarrhea which often accompanies the condition. Bloat also occurs in older cattle (see 4.61).

Differential diagnosis: abomasal dilatation, intestinal torsion.

Management: severe bloat can be relieved by passage of a stomach tube, or in extreme cases by trocar and cannula. Best option may be creation of a semi-permanent rumen fistula. Oral antibiotics will reduce further rumen fermentation, and NSAIDs will relieve the colic. Investigate and improve feeding practices. Suckling from a teat may be preferable to drinking from a bucket in some cases.

Conditions of the skin

Three distinct types of alopecia or hair loss in calves are illustrated.

2

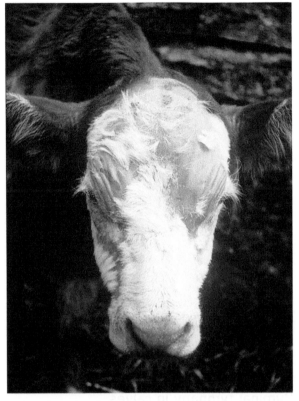

2.39. Idiopathic alopecia (Hereford cross)

Idiopathic alopecia

Spontaneous hair loss often occurs over the head, as in the crossbred Hereford calf (2.39). Less commonly, the whole body may be involved. Milk allergy and vitamin E deficiency are suggested causes. Most cases recover slowly over 1–2 months, without treatment.

Alopecia postdiarrhea

In the Charolais cross calf (2.40), fecal soiling following severe rotavirus scour has totally denuded the perineum and ventral surface of the tail. Following longer bouts of recumbency, there may also be further hair loss over the hock and lower abdomen, including the navel. Urine scald may also be a contributory cause (2.5).

Alopecia of muzzle

Alopecia of this type is seen in calves fed milk substitute, and results from fat globules adhering to the skin over the muzzle. The causes include inadequate mixing of milk substitute, feeding it at too low a temperature, and calves that drink slowly. Hair loss on this 3-week-old crossbred Hereford (2.41) extends from the muzzle onto the nasal arch. The underlying pink skin shows secondary scab formation.

Management: ensure milk substitutes are thoroughly mixed according to manufacturers' instructions, fed at the

2.40. Postdiarrheal alopecia (Charolais cross)

correct temperature, and given to calves that are eager to feed (having been primed by anticipation), thus ensuring that the esophageal groove is functional.

Miscellaneous disorders

Diphtheria (oral necrobacillosis)

Definition: an ulcerative necrosis of the cheek, tongue, pharynx, and larynx caused by *Fusobacterium necrophorum*.

Clinical features: diphtheria can produce a range of clinical signs including painful coughing, dyspnea, and a

2.41. Muzzle alopecia in milk-fed calf (Hereford cross, 3 weeks old)

2.42. Oral necrobacillosis involving cheek (Charolais)

2.43. Oral necrobacillosis showing salivation (Charolais)

fetid odor. The Charolais calf (2.42) is a mild case involving the cheek, and producing an external swelling and oral mucosal ulceration. If the tongue is involved, calves salivate profusely (2.43) and may regurgitate partially masticated food. 2.44 shows a deep ulcerative area at the base of the tongue on the right that has been cleaned to

2.44. Calf diphtheria showing tongue ulceration

2.45. Sublingual erosion in oral necrobacillosis

remove necrotic debris and food, and in another case (2.45) a diphtheritic erosion is visible beneath the tongue.

Differential diagnosis: oral or pharyngeal trauma, actinobacillosis, tooth abscess.

Management: prompt therapy with parenteral antibiotics is usually very effective. Anti-inflammatory drugs may be helpful.

Necrotic laryngitis (laryngeal necrobacillosis)

Definition: a caseo-diphtheritic thickening of the vocal cords caused by *Fusobacterium necrophorum*.

Clinical features: early cases present with stridor ("roaring breathing"), and affected calves are often initially thought to have pneumonia, although the appetite and demeanor remain good and the animal is not pyrexic. More advanced cases develop dyspnea, stand with neck outstretched, and have difficulty feeding owing to severe laryngeal obstruction. Normally, there is no palpable external laryngeal swelling. Contact ulcers of the laryngeal cartilages may be the initial lesions. A fetid odor is often apparent.

Postmortem examination (2.46) reveals a caseous infection (A), typically located bilaterally between the

2.46. Autopsy of laryngeal necrobacillosis

2.47. Laryngeal diphtheria

2.48. Joint ill involving left carpus (Friesian calf)

vocal processes (B) and the medial angles of the arytenoid cartilages (C), where it restricts air passage. In other cases (2.47) the caseous infection may be in the deeper tissues, such as on the left arytenoid area (A) of this 4-month-old Limousin cross calf, where the only superficial change is a soft tissue swelling, the caseous material being deeper within. Note the shape of the normal cartilage (B) on the right.

Differential diagnosis: pharyngeal and laryngeal trauma, severe viral laryngitis (IBR), laryngeal edema or abscessation.

Management: prolonged (e.g., 2–3 weeks) therapy with parenteral antibiotics plus NSAIDs may be effective in early cases. In more advanced cases insertion of a tracheostomy tube under local anesthesia which is left in place for 3–4 weeks (sometimes removed and cleansed daily) to allow the airway to recover, can be reasonably effective.

Joint ill

Definition: non-specific, usually purulent, arthritis of one or more joints of young calves, generally resulting from septicemic spread from navel infection.

Clinical features: septicemic infection entering the navel at birth (see "Navel ill" p. 14) may localize in joints to produce arthritis and severe lameness, especially in colostrum-deficient calves. In the Friesian calf (2.48) the carpus is swollen as a result of intra-articular fibrinopurulent material and a periarticular soft tissue reaction. These changes are seen in the opened carpal joint in 2.49. Advanced cases (2.50) may lead to an open discharge and should be culled well before reaching this stage. Most affected calves are pyrexic. The hock, carpus, and stifle are commonly involved. Polyarthritis is often fatal. Joint ill is first seen at 3–4 weeks old (later than navel ill), and typical cases have no residual evidence of navel infection.

Differential diagnosis: epiphyseal separation (7.122), fractures (7.119).

Management: prompt, aggressive, and prolonged (7–10 days) treatment with broad-spectrum antibiotics, along with anti-inflammatory drugs for a few days. Joint lavage may be useful. Implantation of gentamycin beads or collagen sponges into the joints may give improved results. Response to treatment is generally poor, and many calves are culled when the diagnosis is confirmed.

Iodine deficiency goiter

Clinical features: pregnant cows have an increased iodine requirement, and deficient animals may give birth to stillborn or weakly calves with enlarged thyroids (>20 g), known as goiter. A subcutaneous swelling is clearly visible over the larynx in this 2-week-old Zebu calf from Brazil (2.51), but in the vast majority of cases there

2.49. Joint ill with fibrinopurulent carpitis

2.50. Bilateral carpitis (Italy)

2.52. Bovine neonatal pancytopenia (BNP) in calf (Charolais, 12 days old)

Bovine neonatal pancytopenia (BNP), "bleeding calf syndrome", idiopathic hemorrhagic diathesis

Definition: first reported in 2008, this hemorrhagic diathesis of uncertain etiology is now seen in many EU countries in both dairy and beef herds.

are no external signs and the thyroid glands must be dissected and weighed. Edema and hair loss may also occur. Iodine-deficient soils occur in granite areas, mountainous regions, and areas distant from the sea.

Management: mild cases respond to treatment with iodized salt. Stabilized iodized salt should be fed to dams in all areas suspected to be iodine-deficient, or where the diet contains high levels of goitrogens such as brassicas.

2.53. BNP: extensive small intestinal hemorrhage and intracecal blood clot

2.51. Iodine deficiency goiter in calf (Zebu, 2 weeks old) (Brazil)

2.54. BNP: epicardium, showing multiple confluent hemorrhages

2

Clinical signs: caused by a breakdown of bone marrow erythropoietic cell production. Clinical signs are seen primarily in the first 1–4 weeks of life. These signs include pyrexia and bleeding from various organs including subcutaneous injection and ear-tagging sites, (hence "blood sweating") nose, and rectum. Often a bloody ooze starts from intact skin. Intestinal bleeding may produce melena. Most cases are fatal. In 2.52 a 12-day-old purebred Charolais calf shows skin bleeding at several places including a shoulder injection site, the jugular vein, and nares. It died rapidly, despite supportive therapy. Autopsy of another case showed extensive hemorrhage of the serosal surfaces of the small intestine and a large intracecal blood clot (2.53), while the epicardium was covered with multiple confluent hemorrhages (2.54).

Diagnosis: confirmed on demonstration of the characteristic histopathologic changes of trilineage hypoplasia in the bone marrow. Differential diagnosis: acute coliform septicemia.

Management: supportive therapy only. No specific antidotes are available. A recent (2010) suggestion is that calves from dams which previously have produced a BNP-affected calf should be given only pooled colostrum (i.e., none from the mother).

Chapter 3

Integumentary disorders

Introduction

The skin is the largest organ of the body and performs a wide range of functions. It is mechanically protective against physical injury and provides a barrier against infections, many of which only become established when surface integrity has been compromised by physical or environmental trauma. Sense receptors detect touch and pain. Vitamin D is synthesized under the influence of ultraviolet light. Skin has a primary function in heat control, insulating against heat and cold, and through sweating, it acts as a thermoregulator. The depth and thickness of hair coat is the main factor affecting insulation.

The major breeds of cattle in Europe and North America are derived from *Bos taurus* and have a limited ability to sweat. Cattle derived from *Bos indicus* (Brahman, USA; Africander, Africa), such as the Santa Gertrudis, can sweat copiously for long periods, although there are considerable differences in sweat production from different regions of the body surface.

Visual appraisal of the skin is easily carried out and a wide range of disorders is recognized. Anaphylactic reactions can produce urticaria. Photosensitization may result from a range of intoxications including St. John's Wort, *Lantana*, and facial eczema (see also Chapter 13, 13.13, 13.22–13.24). Parasitic (lice and mange), fungal (ringworm), bacterial infections (skin tuberculosis), and fly infestations (myiasis and warbles) all produce skin changes which are discussed in this chapter. The final section deals with physical conditions such as hematomas, abscesses, frostbite, other traumatic incidents, and neoplasia.

Many skin changes which are secondary to other diseases are described in the relevant chapters, for example, gangrene secondary to mastitis (see 11.8) or ergot poisoning (see 7.159), or subcutaneous swellings associated with urolithiasis (see 10.7) or umbilical (navel) conditions (2.9).

3.1. Cutaneous urticaria in cow (Friesian)

Cutaneous urticaria (urticaria, angioedema, "blaine")

Definition: a vascular reaction of the skin, thought to be an as yet unidentified plant or immunological hypersensitivity, leading to development of multiple wheals.

Clinical features: urticaria is sudden in onset. Cases are sporadic. The wheals do not itch. The Friesian cow (3.1) has raised plaques of edema (wheals) over the face and shoulders. The eyelids and muzzle are swollen. Although looking depressed, she was eating well and, like many such mild cases, recovered within 36 hours. The Simmental cow (3.2) was much more advanced, pyrexic, and in considerable pain. The head, grossly enlarged due to subcutaneous edema, was often rested on the ground. The skin of the muzzle was hyperemic. Localized areas sloughed a few weeks later. Some cases are allegedly due to snake bites or bee stings, but remain unproven.

Differential diagnosis: photosensitization (3.5–3.9).

Management: mild cases resolve spontaneously. More severe cases benefit from rapidly acting corticosteroids, or NSAIDs. There is no known prevention.

3.2. Severe cutaneous urticaria in cow (Simmental)

Photosensitization (photosensitive dermatitis)

Etiology and pathogenesis: photosensitization has a worldwide occurrence. Photoreactive agents accumulating under the skin convert ultraviolet light into thermal energy, leading to inflammatory changes that initially produce skin swelling, and, later, a possible slough. Only white or lightly pigmented skin is affected, since black skin prevents absorption of sunlight. The initial photoreactive agent may have been ingested (primary photosensitization), or may be produced as a result of liver damage (secondary or hepatogenous photosensitization). In cattle the principal secondary photoreactive agents are porphyrins and phylloerythrins, the latter being a normal end product of chlorophyll that is not metabolized further. Liver damage may result from ingestion of a wide range of drugs, plants, or chemicals.

Clinical features: in the early stages, affected animals show marked discomfort and pyrexia, with erythema and encrustation around the margins of the nostrils (3.3) and erythema of the teats (3.4), as in this Simmental cow. The teats are very painful and may later blister and slough (3.5), making milking almost impossible. The thickness

3.3. Photosensitization affecting muzzle margin in cow (Simmental)

3

3.4. Photosensitization with teat erythema in same cow as 3.3

3.5. Photosensitization with sloughing of teat epithelium

of the skin slough, in this case only moderate, depends on the degree of initial damage. The primary febrile phase, edema, and thickening of the white skin had passed unnoticed in the heifer in 3.6, and she was presented with sloughing of dry, hard areas of white skin and with a new epidermis forming beneath. Seven weeks later (3.7) the new skin was well developed. Hair regrowth was possible owing to the preservation of hair follicles deeper in the epidermis. Areas of granulation tissue may retard healing (3.8), especially over bony prominences such as the pelvis. A dry dermatitis persisted in this cow for a further 2 years. The condition also occurs in *Lantana* poisoning (13.13) and facial eczema (13.22–13.24). Serum biochemistry or hepatic biopsy may aid confirmation of liver damage. A more advanced case, involving both udder and teats, is shown in (3.9). The associated pain plus thickening of the teat wall (which prevented the teats filling with milk) made this cow impossible to milk.

Differential diagnosis: BEPP (1.35), foot-and-mouth disease (12.2–12.8), bluetongue (12.17), bovine herpes mammillitis (11.18), vesicular stomatitis (11.26, 11.27). The clinical presentation of early cases, where skin edema may be difficult to detect, strongly resembles colic.

Management: during active photosensitization, cattle should be kept in the shade or preferably housed. Parenteral corticosteroids and NSAIDs may be helpful in early stages to reduce the extent of skin slough. B vitamins may help in cases with hepatic damage. Secondary skin infection and fly strike should be controlled. Skin lesions heal well despite extensive necrosis, leaving residual scarring and wrinkling.

Brown coat color

Copper deficiency affects several systems (see 7.167–7.172), but classically causes loss of coat color. However, copper deficiency is not the only cause of brown coat

3.6. Photosensitization with skin slough and healing in heifer (Friesian)

3.7. Heifer of 3.6, 7 weeks later

3.8. Photosensitization showing healing and granulation tissue in cow (Friesian)

color. Animals turned out to spring grazing may retain their winter coat (3.10), particularly younger animals in poorer body condition and first-lactation heifers. Although grazing the same pasture, the older animal at the rear is not affected.

Differential diagnosis: molybdenum toxicosis (13.34), retention of winter coat associated with ill-thrift.

3.9. Udder sunburn

3.10. Brown coat color, possibly copper deficiency in calves (Hereford cross)

Parasitic skin conditions

Cattle are affected by four genera of mange mites, i.e., *Sarcoptes*, *Chorioptes*, *Psoroptes*, and *Demodex*, six species of lice, skin helminths (*Stephanofilaria* and *Parafilaria*), myiasis (screw-worm), and various fly infestations. In temperate climates parasitic skin infestations are more commonly encountered in housed cattle in winter. Many of the conditions cannot be differentiated on clinical examination alone and laboratory tests are necessary. Often several conditions coexist, e.g., mange, ringworm, and lice commonly occur simultaneously especially on cattle in poorer condition. The appearance and location of mange lesions are generally characteristic for the particular mite, although specific diagnosis depends on microscopic examination of the mouthparts.

Mange

Sarcoptic mange (scabies)

Caused by *Sarcoptes scabiei* var. *bovis*, lesions are typically seen over the head, neck and hindquarters (3.11). Note the hair loss and severe thickening of the skin in 3.12. The white areas show secondary damage due to rubbing. In severe cases there may be almost total hair loss. The close-up view (3.13) shows the dry, scaly appearance of the thickened skin.

Chorioptic mange

Chorioptic mange is the most common type of mange in cattle. The fold of skin beside the tail is the characteristic site for infestation by *Chorioptes bovis* (3.14). Lesions comprise a thick encrustation overlying an area of moist serous exudate. They are intensely irritant. In untreated cases the dry encrustation spreads down the perineum and over the posterior udder. In advanced cases (3.15)

3.11. Sarcoptic mange of head, neck and hind quarters (Friesian)

3.12. Sarcoptic mange of neck and fore quarters (Friesian)

red, pustular lesions may be seen. Less commonly infection is seen in the neck and shoulder region (3.16).

Psoroptic mange

Note the skin thickening and hair loss in the cow (3.17), extending from the vulva to the udder. The condition

3.13. Sarcoptic mange: close-up view of thickened skin

3.14. Chorioptic mange at tail base: acute phase in cow (Friesian)

3.15. Chorioptic mange on perineum

may start at the withers and spread over the whole body. Pruritus is often marked. Psoroptic mange (*Psoroptes ovis*) is notifiable in North America, where eradication programs have been in progress for many years. In recent years psoroptic mange has also become more common in South Wales and elsewhere in Europe, especially Belgium.

3.16. Chorioptic mange on neck

3

3.17.   Psoroptic mange of perineum and udder in cow

Demodectic mange (follicular mange)

Small papules are seen on the white skin of this cow (3.18), from which a thick, white, waxy material containing large numbers of mites can be expressed. Another case (3.19) shows papules over the skin of the shoulder. Some nodules become secondarily infected with *Staphylococci*. The condition is generally mild, with a spontaneous recovery. Extensive hair loss is rare. Similar lesions are seen with *Dermatophilus* (3.38, 3.42).

Management of above forms of mange: as mite eggs take 2–3 weeks to hatch, and as mites can persist in the environment for around 2 weeks, two pour-on organophosphorus treatments, or two subcutaneous injections of ivermectin, 2–3 weeks apart, are needed. Alternative drugs are single doses of doramectin, or eprinomectin, both of which have greater persistence.

3.19.   Demodectic mange: papules and nodules

Psoroptic mange control is problematic. All affected and contact animals should be treated with injectable macrocyclic lactones or licenced pour-on products. But unlicenced products with greater efficacy in the UK are permethrin pour-on or Amitraz, prescribed by a veterinarian, and have potential milk and meat withdrawal disadvantages.

Lice (pediculosis)

Clinical features: sucking lice (e.g., *Haematopinus eurysternus* and *Linognathus vituli* and, in North America, *Solenopotes capillatus*) are slower moving than biting lice (*Damalinia [Bovicola] bovis*). In addition to pruritus (the only lesion due to biting lice), sucking lice may produce severe anemia, loss of condition, and even death. Pediculosis is most prevalent in the winter months. Parting the hair along the back may reveal small, brown, motile lice just visible to the naked eye. They are more easily seen on white skin and hair, or on the hairless skin of the groin (3.20). Note the variation in their size.

Clinically, infestations are manifested by rubbing, biting, scratching, and thickening of the skin. In 3.21 the calf's tongue is protruding and its head is held on one side, a stance typical of pruritus. In early cases the hair develops vertical lines on the neck. Small, hairless areas with white scurf may arise from biting. In more advanced

3.18.   Demodectic mange: papules in cow (Friesian)

3.20.   Lice in inguinal region

3.21. Lice (pediculosis) over shoulder and neck in calf (Friesian cross)

3.22. Lice in neck and beneath mandible in cow (Ayrshire)

cases the skin is thickened round the face and the vertical hair lines on the neck are thrown into thick folds, as in this adult Ayrshire cow (3.22). A further characteristic sign is the presence of clumps of hair (3.23) where affected cattle have been biting their pruritic skin, as opposed to licking and grooming it.

3.23. Raised tufts of hair result from biting to alleviate lice irritation

3.24. Lice eggs ("nits") near ear tag in calf

Younger calves especially may be stunted and anemic, and become much more susceptible to other diseases such as pneumonia, especially with sucking lice infestations. Ringworm often occurs in association with lice: early lesions are seen on the shoulder in 3.21. Pale beige-colored oval lice eggs ("nits"), glued onto the hair shafts, can often be seen with the naked eye, particularly on the ear (3.24 near the tag) and over the shoulders. In older animals the coat may become matted with lice eggs.

Management: lice are most common in conditions of high stocking density, high humidity, a dusty environment, and in colder weather, when the coat becomes thicker. Eggs hatch over a period of 2–3 weeks, and adult lice can persist for around 2 weeks in the environment, so prolonged or repeated treatments are often necessary. Organochlorine compounds, e.g., gamma benzene hexachloride (BHC), are very effective but their use is now prohibited in most countries. Two organophosphorus treatments, 2 weeks apart, can be very effective, e.g., phosmet or coumaphos as a pour-on or as dips, but again their use is restricted in many countries. Permethrin synergized with piperonyl butoxide and tetrachlorvinophos can be used a spray or pour-on. Single pour-on applications of doramectin or eprinectin are also very effective against sucking lice. Badly infested cattle may benefit from multivitamins.

Ringworm (dermatophytosis)

Definition: ringworm is a fungal infection of the superficial, dead, keratinized tissues of the hair and skin. Infection will often track into the hair follicles leading to a temporary alopecia. *Trichophyton verrucosum* is the most common cause in cattle, although occasionally *Microsporum* species may be involved. Ringworm is an important zoonosis.

Clinical features: dermatophytosis is most commonly recognized in calves but is not uncommon in dairy cows,

3

3.25. Ringworm (dermatophytosis) in calf (Friesian)

3.27. Ringworm showing small discrete lesions

especially if they have not previously been exposed to infection. Lesions are commonly seen over the head and neck (3.25), but they may occur on any part of the body. They consist of circular areas of alopecia in which the skin is thickened and often markedly encrusted. The initial stages (3.26) show progressive alopecia and erythema of the skin, with encrustation developing later. Lesions expand from the periphery and several smaller areas may coalesce (3.26). Older animals may show generalized small discrete lesions which are often red in the initial stages (3.27). After hair loss these tend to become erythematous and lack the dry scaly appearance seen in 3.25.

Ringworm causes irritation and if affected calves rub against posts or feed troughs, they deposit spores that can remain infective for up to 4 years.

Management: spontaneous recovery is common. Valuable individual animals may be treated by firstly removal of the encrusted material and then whole body application of a wash or spray of natamycin. Oral dosage with the fungistatic antibiotic griseofulvin is highly effective, but its use is restricted in many countries because of potential concerns about its teratogenic effects. An effective live attenuated vaccine is available.

Skin helminths

Cattle are affected by four genera of skin helminths, *Onchocerca*, *Pelodera* (*Rhabditis bovis*), *Stephanofilaria*, and *Parafilaria*.

Cutaneous stephanofilariasis

Microfilariae of *Stephanofilaria stilesi* are introduced into the skin of the ventral midline by the horn fly (*Haematobia irritans*) as it feeds, producing large, circular areas of dermatitis, seen here on the ventral abdomen (3.28). Recent lesions are moist with blood or serous exudate, whilst long-standing areas are characterized by alopecia and hyperkeratosis.

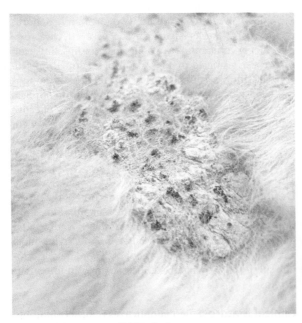

3.26. Ringworm in calf (Friesian)

3.28. Stephanofilariasis in ventral midline of beef cow

3.31. Parafilarial infection in bull (South Africa)

3.29. Stephanofilariasis (parasitic otitis) in cow (Zebu) (India)

Stephanofilarial otitis (parasitic otitis)

Caused by *Stephanofilaria zaheeri*, parasitic otitis is most prevalent in older cattle in humid weather. Note the painful erythematous inflammation on the inside of the ear of this Zebu cow from India (3.29). In East Africa a free-living nematode, *Rhabditis bovis*, can also produce a purulent otitis that may lead to middle ear involvement.

Stephanofilarial dermatitis (hump sore)

Transmitted by flies, *Stephanofilaria assamensis* produces an irritant dermatitis. The raw, granulating area seen on the hump of this crossbred Jersey cow from Bangladesh (3.30) results in lost milk production, reduced working capacity, and hide damage. Exotic cattle are affected more than indigenous breeds.

Parafilarial infection

Clinical features: parafilarial infection is common in parts of Asia, Africa, and Europe, including the UK. Transmitted by flies of the *Musca* genus, *Parafilaria bovicola* produces painful subcutaneous lesions that may reduce the productivity of draught animals, but, more importantly, can lead to serious economic losses from carcass trimming of beef cattle at slaughter. The female worm perforates the host's skin and oviposits into blood dripping from the wound. A typical "bleeding spot" is illustrated on the chest wall of this South African bull (3.31). (The fecal soiling on the crest wall of the neck is coincidental.) Flies feeding on the blood, which may continue to flow for several hours, ingest eggs containing microfilariae. A typical female worm nodule is shown in 3.32, closely adherent to the hide.

Management: fly control, including dipping and impregnated ear tags, is important in prevention.

Besnoitiosis

Definition: besnoitiosis is a protozoon disease of cattle caused by the cyst-forming apicomplexan parasite *Besnoitia besnoiti*, with two forms: an acute, mild, or inapparent clinical disease, and a later severe, debilitating, but not usually fatal stage. The disease was reported originally in Sub-Saharan Africa, the Middle East, Asia, and South America. In February 2010 it was classed as an "emerging disease" in Europe, which for decades had only sporadic

3.30. Stephanofilariasis dermatitis (hump sore) in cow (Jersey cross) (Bangladesh)

3.32. Typical *Parafilaria bovicola*: female worm in subcutis (South Africa)

3

3.33. Besnoitiosis in bull (South Africa)

3.35. Subscleral nodules in besnoitiosis (Limousin, Germany)

cases in southern Portugal and along the French–Spanish Pyrenean border. Now reported elsewhere in Spain, Italy, Portugal, France, and Germany, its mode of transmission is uncertain, but is probably by insects. Spread in Europe is possibly by international trade of subclinically infected breeding stock.

Clinical features: in the acute first stage clinical signs may include dyspnea, anorexia, pyrexia (possible abortion) and weight loss, though the majority of cases are asymptomatic. At the same time some cattle develop minute, pinhead-sized, whitish subscleral nodules, parasitic cysts (3.35), which may later also be visible to a lesser extent in the vulval submucosa (3.36). In the second stage skin changes start with ventral (also udder and teats) and limb edema (anasarca) followed by progressive thickening and wrinkling of the skin, alopecia, hyperkeratosis, and typical scleroderma (3.33, 3.34). A South African bull (3.33) with chronic sclerodermatitis ("elephant skin") has marked (2 cm) thickening of the skin and complete hair loss over such areas. The skin may crack (3.34) over exposed areas following mild trauma, resulting in secondary infection and possible myiasis. Signs tend to appear in the summer months associated with fly activity. The current economic importance of besnoitiosis in Europe

has not been accurately estimated. Diagnosis depends on demonstration of typical cysts (via skin biopsy), or by various laboratory techniques in infected but asymptomatic cattle (e.g. ELISA, IFAT).

Differential diagnosis: in acute form: bluetongue (p. 225), malignant catarrhal fever (p. 226), and BVD-MD (p. 54); in chronic sclerodermal stage: sarcoptic mange, mycosis, thermal burns, photosensitivity, cutaneous lymphosarcoma, hyperkeratosis, dermatophilosis.

Management: quarantine of all purchased stock is recommended, elimination of infected animals, avoidance of iatrogenic transmission, and insect control. No effective vaccines or drugs are available in Europe.

Other bacterial and viral skin disorders

Dermatophilosis (cutaneous streptothricosis)

Definition: skin lesions caused by infection with the actinomycete *Dermatophilus congolensis*, and sometimes

3.34. Scleroderma on hock wound evident (Portugal)

3.36. Submucosal vulval nodules (Limousin, Germany)

3.37. Dermatophilosis affecting whole cow

3.38. Dermatophilosis (cutaneous streptothricosis) on hindquarters of cow

3.39. Dermatophilosis in calf

erroneously called "mycotic dermatitis" following exposure to prolonged periods of wet weather (also called "rain rot" or "rain scald").

Clinical features: in temperate climates lesions are mild, as in the Friesian cow 3.37, which has nonpruritic, raised clumps of hair (which can be easily lifted off) with a light-brown, waxy exudate at the base. A close-up view of another cow is shown in 3.38. Damp areas of skin arising from spillage of milk can result in significant *Dermatophilus* lesions developing around the muzzle, chin and ventral neck regions of milk-fed calves (3.39). Severely affected suckler calves may die from reduced feed intakes, especially if the teats of the dam are affected (3.40). A closer view of thickened coat and skin in the hock areas, from another case is seen in (3.41). In warmer climates, particularly during periods of high humidity and increased fly and tick activity, zoospores dormant in the epidermis may become active in almost epidemic proportions to cause more severe skin damage, with secondary inflammation. This cow from Antigua (3.42) shows small, raised, nodular skin tufts, especially over the neck and shoulders. More advanced lesions coalesce to form plaques (3.43, also West Indian origin) with an almost

3.40. Dermatophilosis of teat

3.41. Dermatophilosis of hock, close up

3.42. Dermatophilosis in cow (Antigua, West Indies)

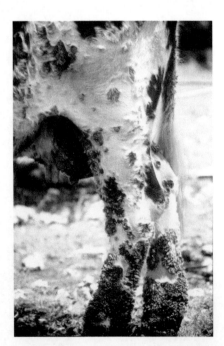

3.43. Dermatophilosis, advanced, on hind legs (West Indies)

wart-like appearance. Chronic severe cases can lead to emaciation.

Differential diagnosis: warble fly (3.50, 3.51), lumpy-skin disease (12.24), mud fever (7.66), parakeratosis in calves (1.28).

Management: housed cattle can be provided with self-grooming facilities such as wall brushes. Provide shelter from rain and avoid skin trauma and damp conditions. Severe cases may benefit from parenteral antibiotics (penicillin) and multivitamins.

Fibropapillomatosis (papillomatosis, warts)

Clinical features: warts, predominantly seen in 6–18-month-old cattle, appear as fleshy lumps on the head and neck. Large, pendulous warts may also be seen along the brisket and sternum. Their size varies enormously, from 5 cm in diameter (3.44) to small nodules, only just visible above the hair of the skin. They sometimes occur in the neck region of adult draught cattle, seen here in an Egyptian native Baladi cow (3.45). Warts also occur on teats (11.29–11.31), penis (10.19), and in the bladder (13.4), where they are associated with bracken poisoning. Skin warts are caused by papovaviruses. Five species have been reported, including three distinct species on teats. Warts are most commonly seen in larger groups of young cattle. Flies and lice may be important in transmission.

Management: most warts, even penile lesions, resolve spontaneously with age following development of viral immunity. Pedunculated warts may often be pulled off, sometimes following ligation of the pedicle. Some success has been claimed for simple autogenous vaccines. Extensive accumulation of warts may trap debris and develop secondary infection. These benefit from washing and superficial disinfection.

3.44. Fibropapillomatosis (warts)

3.45. Fibropapillomatosis in neck region of cow (Baladi) (Egypt)

Skin tuberculosis (atypical mycotuberculosis)

Definition: indurated nodules, running along the path of corded lymphatics beneath the skin, contain nonpathogenic, acid-fast bacteria which may affect the reaction to the tuberculin skin test for TB.

Clinical features: These subcutaneous nodules are most commonly seen on the legs, neck, and shoulder region (3.46). Their subcutaneous position (at least six are evident) makes them easy to distinguish from the intradermal nodular reaction to tuberculin. Some consider these chains of subcutaneous nodules are typical for animals infected with bovine immunodeficiency virus (BIV) but this is unlikely.

Management: no control necessary. Note significance in TB testing.

3.46. Skin tuberculosis in cow (Friesian, Netherlands)

3.47. Nocardiosis ("farcy")

Lymphangitis, lymphadenitis, and bovine farcy

Clinical features: in dairy cows the most common form of lymphadenitis (inflammation of lymph nodes) and lymphangitis (lymph ducts) is associated with an ascending infection of the lower limb following the line of the lymphatics. In 3.47 a series of small abscesses are visible along the line of the lymphatics, some of which (A) have ulcerated ("ulcerative lymphangitis"), and others (B) are seen as discrete soft fluctuating swellings. Environmental organisms such as *Arcanobacterium pyogenes* are commonly involved, and the animal may be mildly pyrexic in the early stages. Bovine farcy is a purulent lymphangitis and lymphadenitis caused by *Nocardia farcinica*.

Differential diagnosis: skin tuberculosis (3.46), ulcerative lymphadenitis (3.48), skin lymphosarcoma (12.77), lumpy skin disease (12.24), dermatophilosis (3.37–3.43).

Management: antibiotic therapy will resolve mild cases, but not bovine farcy.

Ulcerative lymphangitis (caseous lymphadenitis: pseudotuberculosis)

Caused by *Corynebacterium pseudotuberculosis*, ulcerative lymphangitis is primarily a condition of sheep and goats, although cattle can very occasionally be affected.

3.48. Ulcerative lymphangitis (pseudotuberculosis) in left foreleg of cow (Friesian) (USA)

The large nodules seen in the foreleg and elbow in 3.48 probably involve drainage lymph nodes of the lymphatics. When spontaneous rupture occurs, the ulcerated lymphangitis lesions typically release a caseous material heavily infected with *C. pseudotuberculosis*.

Differential diagnosis: skin tuberculosis (3.46), lymphangitis (3.47).

Management: cull, as attempts at resolution via drainage and prolonged irrigation are rarely successful, and contamination of environment presents a potent risk of infection.

Fly infestations

A wide range of fly species feed on cattle, the most common being horn flies, buffalo flies (*Haematobia irritans* spp.) seen on the skin of the back in 3.49, head flies (*Hydrotoea irritans*) and face flies (*Musca autumnalis*). These flies preferentially congregate on the withers, flanks, and around the eyes. In addition to causing annoyance, and therefore restricting feed intake, these flies may also produce anemia and transmit disease, for example, *Parafilaria* and *Moraxella bovis* in infectious bovine keratoconjunctivitis (IBK).

Management: insecticide sprays, back rubbers, traps.

Warble fly ("warbles")

Definition: warble fly or "warbles" comprises a range of syndromes caused by migrating larvae of *Hypoderma*

3.49. Head fly (*H. irritans*) infestation over back

and *Dermatobia* species. Skin damage is most common, but spinal paralysis, choke from esophageal inflammation, generalized illness from mass migration of larvae, and anaphylactic reactions can also occur.

Clinical features: there are two species of warble fly (heel fly): *Hypoderma bovis* and *H. lineatum*. Both lay eggs on the hair of the lower legs. Emerging larvae penetrate the epidermis and migrate subcutaneously to the skin of the back, which they puncture for breathing holes, and then encyst. Encysted larvae in the subdermal tissues produce smooth skin swellings (3.50) known as warbles. Over a period of 4–6 weeks, warble larvae undergo three molts, the light-cream to dark-brown third-stage larvae then emerging through the breathing hole to fall to the ground to pupate. In 3.51 a late third-stage larva has been manually expressed onto the skin, over the anterior chest. A cluster of five larval breathing holes, with larvae feeding beneath, is present in the skin, dorsal to the lumbar

3.50. Warble fly infestation showing several encysted subcutaneous larvae

3.51. Warbles along back of cow (Friesian)

3.53. Tropical warble fly infestation in cow (Hereford cross) (Brazil)

spine. Losses due to warbles arise from damage to the most valuable part of the hide, from reduced grazing due to fear of the adult fly, and rare cases of paralysis resulting from hypersensitivity to dead larvae in the spinal canal.

Management: systemic insecticides, e.g., organophosphorus compounds (contraindicated in lactating cattle) or avermectins. Warble fly infestation is a notifiable disease in many countries, including the UK, where it has been eradicated, and specific control measures must be followed.

Tropical warble fly: *Dermatobia hominis*

Clinical features: *Dermatobia hominis* is known as the tropical warble fly. It is distributed only between southern Mexico and Argentina in South America, where it is a major problem. Human infection can also occur. The adult lays its eggs on a range of other insects (49 different species have been recorded), which then transmit the eggs to cattle when feeding on them. Eggs are visible between the wings of the fly, *Musca domestica*, in 3.52. On hatching, larvae rapidly burrow through the skin and

encyst to form a subcutaneous nodule, the warble. Firm *Dermatobia* warble nodules are seen on the Hereford crossbred cow from Brazil (3.53), especially over the shoulders and flanks. (Warbles of *Hypoderma* are seen only along the back, 3.51.) After feeding for 40–50 days, the mature larvae emerge (3.54) and fall to the ground to pupate. Severe pain and irritation, with secondary infection, may occur as the larvae emerge, as seen in the Zebu cow in 3.55.

Management: as for warble fly; some cattle strains show resistance to *D. hominis*.

Screw-worm or myiasis

Clinical features: the parasites known as screw-worms are the larvae of the blowflies *Cochliomyia hominivorax* and *Chrysomyia bezziana*. The adult fly lays eggs on wounds, the navel of neonates, or on tick-damaged areas (12.34). 3.56 shows an early infestation. More advanced

3.52. Tropical warble fly egg infestation on fly (Brazil)

3.54. Mature warble larvae emerging through skin (Brazil)

3

3.55. Secondary infection in warble infestation in cow (Zebu) (Brazil)

lesions (3.57) may be filled with larvae of mixed ages, some of which will be mature and ready to leave and pupate in the soil. A profuse, foul-smelling exudate with extensive skin damage is typical. The disease is of major importance in South America and has been reported in North Africa and Southern Asia.

Differential diagnosis: vital to differentiate screwworm from other fly larvae. Mature larvae are pink, 1–2 cm long and have rows of fine dark spines on the anterior part of each segment. Transport to laboratory in 70% alcohol for identification.

3.56. Screw-worm infestation (myiasis) showing blow-fly eggs in wound (Brazil)

3.57. Myiasis, more advanced, showing eggs and larvae (Brazil)

Management: notifiable disease in some countries which have eradication campaigns. Local and systemic (spray, dip) treatment with organophosphorus compounds and avermectins.

Traumatic and physical conditions

In addition to being the largest organ of the body, the skin is also the most exposed. Injury is common, particularly when cattle, housed in poorly designed, overcrowded buildings are handled roughly. Failure to dehorn housed cattle predisposes to further injury. Damp, dirty conditions may compromise the skin defenses. When such factors are combined with inadequate bedding and projections from housing, abscesses or more severe injuries can result. Cattle can withstand wide extremes of temperature, although frostbite does occur. Hematomas are commonly the result of physical injury, whilst other subcutaneous swellings may result from hernia, abscesses, or rupture.

Hematoma

Clinical features: hematomas are initially soft, painless, fluctuating, fluid-filled swellings that appear suddenly. Common sites are points with no muscle cover where skin trauma against bone can occur, e.g., over the pelvic prominences shown here at the tuber ischii (3.58), over the spine (3.59), the lower flank (3.60), and the shoulder. Occasionally hematomas spread into the pelvic cavity, increasing intrapelvic pressure and interfering with urination and defecation. The case in 3.59 occurred as a result of being trapped under a cubicle (free stall) division, and the flank hematoma (3.60) followed a horn gore. Without rupturing, the majority of smaller hematomas resolve to leave thick skin folds, seen in 3.61, which followed the resolution of a hematoma over the

3.58. Hematoma over ischial tuberosity in cow (Ayrshire)

3.59. Large hematoma over spine in cow (Friesian)

tuber ischii. Sometimes a hematoma becomes infected and develops into an abscess. In 3.62 two small abscesses, both originating from hematomas, are clearly seen to the right of the tail head overlying the tuber ischii. Occasionally, hematomas burst, releasing the blood clot.

Differential diagnosis: abscess, flank rupture, hernia.

3.60. Flank hematoma in cow (Friesian)

3.61. Skin folds in healing hematoma

Management: minimal interference is best for most cases, as spontaneous resolution occurs. Some hematomas develop into abscesses and need drainage. Occasional cases are so extensive that culling is necessary.

Prevention: identify, then minimize, points of trauma.

Rib fracture

Clinical features: older cows, and especially chronically lame cows, commonly develop a fracture of the eighth and ninth rib, specifically at the costochondral junction, which is a true arthrodesis joint. This is seen externally as a hard swelling approximately one hand breadth behind the point of the elbow (3.63). In other cases the affected rib may be displaced longitudinally, with its caudal edge protruding. A radiograph of this cow (3.64) demonstrates that, compared with the joint on the left, three costochondral joints are damaged, especially the central one, which has a bone spicule dislodged to the right of the joint. Fractures are also visible on the cartilaginous floating ribs. As these calcify with age (i.e., they are not osseous tissue), they do not heal and continued movement at the fracture site causes pain. It has been postulated that rib fracture is one reason why lame cows walk with an arched back, as the fracture site must cause pain, and in some cows a pain response can be elicited on palpation. One suggested cause is that, when

3.62. Two small hematomas to the right of the tail head have developed into abscesses

3

3.63. Rib fracture (costochondral)

lying down, lame cows drop more heavily onto the ground surface than normal cows. The subsequent dorsoventral compression of the chest leads to fracture at the weakest points, which are the costochondral junctions and floating ribs. At a different site, midshaft fractures affecting ribs two to four (under the scapula) are not uncommon at slaughter but are thought to have a different etiology.

Management: minor lesions that are palpable only and not visible require no treatment. As severe lesions lead to locomotor difficulties, affected cows should be housed in straw yards and not in free stalls. If a high herd incidence is seen, factors causing lameness should be investigated.

Bursitis of the neck

Clinical features: in 3.65, hair loss at the cranial aspect of the neck lesion indicates that the bursitis was caused by continually pushing against a feed barrier. Like a hematoma, the swelling is soft, painless, and fluctuating, but it develops more slowly. Aspiration disclosed a clear

3.65. Bursitis of dorsal neck region in cow (Friesian)

fluid. Bursitis also occurs on the hock (7.132) and carpus (7.147) as a result of inadequately bedded free stalls.

Management: individual lesions are best left to resolve spontaneously, having first removed the animal from the source of trauma. If several cattle are affected, then structural changes may be indicated, e.g., improving free stall bedding and comfort.

Skin abscesses

Clinical features: abscesses are generally hard, hot, and slightly painful swellings that develop and enlarge slowly, thus differentiating them from a hematoma (3.58) or a hernia (3.70), which usually appear suddenly. The Hereford steer (3.66) has a sterile abscess on its neck, caused by the injection of a vaccine. Injecting a 40% solution of calcium borogluconate subcutaneously can lead to a hard, fluid-filled, sterile swelling developing over a period of 3–6 weeks. The popliteal region is a common site for abscessation, as seen in the Friesian cow (3.67). A large, fluctuating swelling is seen on the left leg, lateral to

3.64. Radiograph of rib fractures

3.66. Sterile abscess in steer (vaccine) (Hereford)

3.67.   Abscess in popliteal region in cow (Friesian)

the stifle. The abscess is often situated deep in the muscle and may slowly enlarge over several months.

Although use of the mammary vein for intravenous injection, e.g., for hypocalcemia, is easy for the operator, it carries an increased risk of abscessation (3.68) due to its dependent position and risk of postinjection hemorrhage, especially if nonsterile equipment (e.g., needle) is used. A rare condition, a fibroma (3.69) may also be confused with a mammary abscess, although it will be slow-growing, pendulant, firm, and nonfluctuating on palpation.

Management: abscesses are best left to develop until one part of the capsule is obviously softer, and then lanced at this point, drained, and flushed to achieve resolution. Repeated pressure irrigation is also useful. Great care is required in the confirmation of mammary abscesses.

3.69.   Midline fibroma

Flank hernia

Clinical features: the flank hernia in the Hereford cow (3.70) had developed suddenly, probably as a result of a head butt by another cow, 2 months before presentation. Other cases occur spontaneously, especially in older cows in late pregnancy, where pressure of intra-abdominal contents will be a predisposing factor.

Differential diagnosis: swellings in this area can be difficult to distinguish between an abscess, hematoma, flank hernia, and rupture of the prepubic tendon or anterior udder ligament. With the cow in lateral recumbency, it should be possible to replace the contents of a hernia into the abdomen. This is not possible with other swellings in this position.

Management: large flank hernias in adult cattle can rarely be successfully treated by surgery, and tend to enlarge in late pregnancy, reducing in size after calving when the cow is best culled.

Rupture of prepubic tendon

The udder has dropped ventrally, and the sac of skin and muscle anterior to it contains abdominal organs (3.71).

3.68.   Mammary vein abscess

3.70.   Flank hernia in cow (Hereford)

3

3.71. Rupture of prepubic tendon in cow (Friesian)

Hydrallantois had resulted in the excessive abdominal distension and subsequent rupture.

Differential diagnosis: Flank hernia (p. 47).

Management: repair is hopeless, and culling is indicated if the cow is adversely affected.

Infected ear tag

Clinical features: infection of an ear tag occurs as a result of poor hygiene at insertion, when insufficient space is allowed for growth of the ear margin, or when the tag is inserted too close to the ear base. In 3.72 granulation tissue and a wet, purulent exudate have developed around the tag. Such areas are painful and subject to myiasis.

Management: the tag must be removed and the area cleansed, whereupon the residual wound heals rapidly. The replacement tag must be inserted into a different area.

3.73. Ear necrosis following neonatal frostbite (Limousin)

Ear necrosis from frostbite

The tips of both ears of the Limousin cow (3.73) are missing: the cause was neonatal frostbite. Scrotal frostbite is illustrated in 10.38.

Differential diagnosis: septicemia, typically associated with peracute salmonellosis (2.22), fescue toxicity (7.158), and ergot poisoning (7.159) can produce similar changes in the extremities.

Skin necrosis following caustic dehorning paste

Excessive use of caustic dehorning paste produced the scab-covered skin slough extending from the horn bud towards the eye of this Limousin calf (3.74).

3.72. Infected ear tag site

3.74. Skin necrosis of head due to caustic dehorning paste

3.75. Burns along back, flank and chest wall

Skin burns

Cattle exposed to fire and heat will commonly stand close together in a group with their heads away from the source of danger. Note the scorched skin over the back, upper flanks, and chest of this Holstein cow (3.75), one of a group of 35 dry cows trapped in a yard beside a stack of blazing straw. Although the majority recovered, burns to the udder and teats (visible on the front right teat) meant that many were impossible to milk and had to be culled after calving.

Management: anti-inflammatory drugs may reduce inflammation in the early stages. The possibility of early culling should be considered if an insurance claim is involved.

Ingrowing horn

Etiology and pathogenesis: the horn tip in 3.76, which has now been removed, had penetrated through the skin into the underlying dermis, producing this painful, festering wound, which could develop secondary myiasis. In extreme cases the horn tip may penetrate the skull. This has serious welfare implications. Although some cases develop as a result of apparently normal horn growth in older cattle, the majority are the result of earlier horn damage.

3.76. Ingrowing horn: skin damage

3.77. Tail tip necrosis

Management: check the space between horn tip and skin in any suspect case. The horn tip is nonsensitive and can be removed without local anesthetic.

Tail-tip necrosis

Clinical features: tail-tip necrosis (3.77) is seen as a group problem in steers, heifers, and beef bulls in overcrowded accommodation with slatted floors. The typical tail-tip damage is seen close-up in 3.77. The tip is trampled causing initial trauma followed by suppuration with the risk of ascending infection and septicemic spread to other organs. Tail necrosis in a beef bull (3.78) resulted in an ascending *Arcanobacterium pyogenes* infection, and involvement of the proximal coccygeal nerve supply has resulted in tail paralysis. Risk factors include slatted concrete floors, close confinement, and humid conditions. The tail is repeatedly trapped between the hock and floor

3.78. Tail tip necrosis in beef bull

as the animal makes several attempts to stand. Individual cases may be seen in dairy cows where the injuries typically arise from tails becoming trapped in automatic passage scrapers, the diagonal bars of gates, or trauma from rough handling during restraint. Diagnosis is easy.

Management: affected animals should be detected early and undergo amputation of the tail, with antibiotic therapy.

Prevention: appropriate husbandry and housing changes to reduce injury and overcrowding, and improved bedding.

Tail sequestrum

Clinical features: tail fractures can occur as the result of rough handling or trauma, e.g., when a tail is stood on by another cow in overcrowded yards, or occasionally, when it is caught in a gate or similar structure. Simple fractures result in a deviation of the tail at the point of fracture and appear to cause little discomfort. Complicated fractures and those involving a bony sequestrum often result in a chronic discharging sinus and discomfort, as in 3.79.

Management: amputation is the only treatment option.

Fecolith

Etiology and pathogenesis: fecoliths (hard accumulations of dry feces on the tail, developing during bouts of diarrhea) can occur spontaneously, or may develop around tail marker tape. The drying fecal mass

3.80. Fecolith causing tail damage

contracts, constricts the blood flow and produces swelling and ulceration, as seen on the left of the fecolith in 3.80. When removed, the full extent of the ischemic necrosis is apparent (3.81). The tail tip eventually sloughed. Similar injuries can be caused by incorrectly applied marker tape.

Management: fecoliths are most easily removed by first cracking open the dry fecal ring between two hard surfaces, e.g., with gentle use of a hammer. Tail tape should be removed when no longer needed.

Skin tumors

Horn core carcinoma

Definition: a squamous cell carcinoma of the mucosa of the frontal sinus, developing in horned or

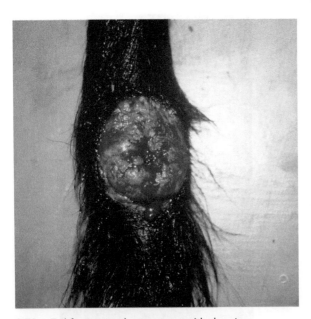

3.79. Tail fracture and sequestrum with chronic discharging sinus

3.81. Ischemic necrosis seen after fecolith removal from 3.80

3.82. Horn core carcinoma in cow (Holstein, 6 years old)

3.83. Melanoma on hock (Charolais cross, 3 weeks old)

dehorned breeds, is especially common in the Indian subcontinent.

Clinical features: a severe case of horn core cancer is shown in 3.82, a 6-year-old Holstein cow in the UK, which had been dehorned at 2 years old. The tumor grew slowly at first, was worried by flies, and suddenly showed this massive enlargement. The frontal sinus was filled with neoplastic and granulation tissue. Metastases were present in regional nodes.

Differential diagnosis: early stages may resemble a frontal sinusitis.

Management: incurable.

Melanocytoma (melanoma)

Definition: sporadic bovine tumor arising from melanocytes in the skin or subcutis, often in younger cattle, occasionally congenital.

Clinical features: this discrete benign melanoma on the left hock of a 3-week-old Charolais crossbred heifer (3.83) was present at birth. It is lobulated, extending both medially and laterally. Gray or black and painless, it presents an obvious cosmetic blemish.

Management: many are amenable to surgery, such as this case, which did not recur in the succeeding 2 years.

Alimentary disorders

Introduction

Chapter 4 illustrates those conditions with primary alimentary signs. It excludes congenital (e.g., cleft palate) and acquired neonatal conditions (e.g., calfhood enteritis). The first section comprises infectious and contagious diseases: bovine virus diarrhea/mucosal disease (BVD/MD) complex, vesicular stomatitis, papular stomatitis (all of which have rather similar gross features), and paratuberculosis. The second section covers the alimentary parasitic conditions: ostertagiasis, and small and large intestinal parasitism (for coccidiosis, see 2.31, 2.32). The remaining conditions are listed by anatomical site (oral cavity to anus), irrespective of their traumatic, nutritional, or other etiology.

Viral diseases

Three viral diseases present problems clinically in differential diagnosis: bovine virus diarrhea/mucosal disease (BVD/MD), vesicular stomatitis, and bovine papular stomatitis. In some regions, further differential diagnosis from foot-and-mouth disease and rinderpest may be necessary (see 12.2–12.15). The pathogenicity and economic importance of these vesicular viral diseases vary greatly. Accurate differentiation is essential and usually depends on laboratory studies.

Bovine virus diarrhea/mucosal disease (BVD/MD)

Definition: major infectious disease caused by a pestivirus.

Clinical features: BVD/MD is a major viral disease worldwide. Congenital defects such as cerebellar hypoplasia and cataracts (8.1, 8.4) may develop in the progeny of females infected during early pregnancy. BVD/MD causes diarrhea and unthriftiness in young cattle. Erosive stomatitis and rhinitis occur, together with similar lesions on other mucous membranes.

In utero infection in the first trimester can produce early embryonic death and infertility, and in the early to mid-fetal period congenital abnormalities such as cerebellar hypoplasia or, less commonly, hydranencephaly, as in the Piedmontese calf in 4.1. Though alert, and suckling with difficulty, it was unable to stand. It was relatively normal at rest, but extensor spasm and opisthotonus developed on minimal stimulation, e.g., when attempting to feed. Cerebellar hypoplasia was confirmed at autopsy examination. 4.2 shows a normal brain (left) and the affected brain (following infection of the dam at 150 days' gestation).

4.2. Normal (left) and hypoplastic cerebellum in BVD/MD

In utero infection in the second trimester, before the age of immunological competence of the fetus, can lead to the birth of a persistently infected calf which is BVD antigen positive, but antibody negative. Such animals may be either clinically normal or stunted, but they continually excrete virus. Unpredictable nervous signs such as aggression may be seen in some BVD persistent infection (P1) calves. At a later date, usually 3–30 months old, superinfection with a noncytopathic strain of BVD virus leads to a syndrome of mucosal disease, with ulceration throughout the gastrointestinal tract. Clinically these animals present signs of oral, intestinal and respiratory involvement. Erosions and hyperemia around the nares, lips, and gums are seen in 4.3.

The specimen in 4.4 shows numerous erosive and hemorrhagic lesions over the entire hard palate. Secondary bacterial infection of the lesions produces the necrotic ulcers seen in the caudal pharynx and rima glottidis

4.1. Cerebellar hypoplasia in BVD/MD in calf (Piedmontese)

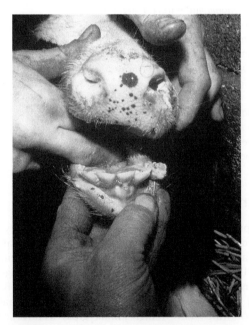

4.3. Bovine virus diarrhea calf with muzzle and oral hyperemic changes

4.4. BVD showing erosive changes in hard palate

4.6. BVD with abomasal hemorrhage and erosions at autopsy

(4.5). Necrosis and abscessation surround the epiglottis. The laryngeal mucosa is also hemorrhagic. Pus lies between the arytenoids, making respiratory efforts difficult and painful. Similar necrotic ulcers may extend over the hard palate, down the esophagus and into the abomasum. The esophagus may have patchy, linear areas of hemorrhage, edema and erosions. Erosions may be seen on the edematous and hyperemic edges of the abomasal rugae (4.6). Small intestinal erosions can lead to mucosal sloughing and the production of casts that pack the intestinal lumen (4.7). A secondary bacterial infection may be responsible for the enlarged nodes. Erosions may also occur around the coronary band and in the interdigital cleft (4.8).

The two cattle in 4.9 are both 18 months old. The nearer heifer, with an abnormal, rust-colored coat, is stunted as a result of chronic, persistent infection (antigen positive, antibody negative) due to maternal infection with BVD virus acquired in early pregnancy. Many of the

4.7. Intestinal mucosal casts in BVD

mucosal changes are so severe as to leave the chronic, persistent infective case emaciated (as in the crossbred animal in 4.10) and a constant source of infection to susceptible contact cattle.

In some herds primary BVD in nonimmune cattle can also produce severe enteric signs and an increased

4.5. BVD with severe changes in caudal pharynx and larynx

4.8. Erosions at coronary band in BVD

4.11.   Vesicular stomatitis: pale lesions on hard palate, dental pad and gums in calf (Charolais)

Vesicular stomatitis

Definition: caused by a rhabdovirus (two strains: New Jersey and Indiana) causing vesicular formation in various superficial tissues. It is probably spread by insect vectors.

Clinical features: the Charolais calf shows blanched areas on the rugae of the hard palate, dental pad, and gums (4.11). These pale areas are vesicles that rupture after some days (4.12). Secondary infection is rare. Vesicular stomatitis has only been confirmed in North and South America. Many animals may be simultaneously affected on one farm, showing excessive salivation, together with oral and possibly teat lesions. Teat lesions (11.26) in vesicular stomatitis can cause problems with milking. Secondary lesions may involve the claws.

4.9.   BVD/MD: nearer rust-colored stunted calf with chronic persistent infection (18 months old)

mortality, especially in dairy cows, although most primary infections in younger animals are subclinical.

Differential diagnosis: salmonellosis, paratuberculosis (4.16), winter dysentery (4.19, 4.20) and other causes of acute enteritis in individuals. Bovine papular stomatitis (4.13), vesicular stomatitis (4.12), FMD (12.2–12.8) and other causes of oral ulceration.

Management: long-term program needed for effective control: persistently infected virus-positive cattle should be identified by blood-testing and culled, as they represent the major source of virus. Screen all purchased stock. Double-fence neighboring cattle. Vaccinate prior to service to prevent the development of persistently infected offspring.

Differential   diagnosis: foot-and-mouth   disease (12.2–12.8) and bovine papular stomatitis (4.13, 4.14). Diagnosis by ELISA or CF test, and if negative, following passage, virus neutralization tests.

Management: suspect cases should be immediately reported to State authorities. (Transboundary disease of Office International des Épizooties (OIE).)

4.10.   BVD/MD: chronic emaciated crossbred steer

4.12.   Vesicular stomatitis: recently ruptured vesicles on hard palate

4.13. Bovine papular stomatitis: papules on muzzle and around nares

4.15. Bovine papular stomatitis

Bovine papular stomatitis (BPS)

Definition: mild disease caused by a parapox virus classified as a "paravaccinia virus" which generally has no adverse effect on the calf.

Clinical features: shallow papules and vesicles are seen on the muzzle, hard palate and gums of these young cattle (4.13, 4.14). Papules develop a distinct roughened center that sometimes expands to merge with adjacent vesicles. A Hereford crossbred calf (4.15) also shows muzzle and nares with ruptured vesicles. Teats are not affected. Immature cattle, sometimes an entire group, are usually involved and recovery is rapid. Systemic effects are rare.

Differential diagnosis: foot-and-mouth disease (12.2–12.8) and vesicular stomatitis (4.11, 4.12).

Management: specific treatment is rarely necessary.

Johne's disease (paratuberculosis)

Definition: chronic wasting disease caused by *Mycobacterium avium paratuberculosis* (formerly *M. johnei*).

Clinical features: Johne's disease causes progressive weight loss, leading to eventual emaciation, although animals may remain alert and continue to eat. This chronic wasting disease is characterized by a profuse, watery diarrhea as seen in an 8-year-old Santa Gertrudis cow (4.16). Clinical signs of wasting and watery diarrhea are evident in a 2-year-old Blonde d'Aquitaine bull (4.17). When compared with normal ileum (4.18), the mucosa in a clinically overt case (A) shows numerous, thick, transverse rugae that cannot be smoothed out by stretching. Local intestinal lymph nodes are usually enlarged and pale, and may contain granulomatous areas. The usual age range is 3–9 years for the onset of clinical signs, which may be insidious, or develop suddenly after calving. Carrier animals excrete for many months prior to this. Infection is introduced into healthy herds by subclinical carriers. Young calves become infected *in utero*, via colostrum, or by oral ingestion. Age immunity develops by 4–6 months old.

4.14. Bovine papular stomatitis: vesicles developing on gums

4.16. Johne's disease showing severe diarrhea in cow (Santa Gertrudis, 8 years old)

4

4.17. Johne's disease (paratuberculosis): severe diarrhea (see tail) in bull (Blonde d'Aquitaine, 2 years old)

The disease may be potentially zoonotic (Crohn's disease).

Differential diagnosis: salmonellosis, severe parasitism, BVD.

Management: no effective treatment is known. Suspect cows should be tested (ELISA, CF, AGID), and culled if positive. Biopsy and histopathology of intestinal lymph nodes is an effective method of diagnosis. Vaccines have limited efficacy in control. There is no test to detect accurately subclinical carriers, and heifers from infected dams should be culled. Reduce spread of infection by hygiene at calving and possibly by pasteurization of pooled colostrum. Separate newly–born calves from their potentially infected dams at once.

Winter dysentery (winter diarrhea)

Definition: etiology uncertain, although coronavirus has recently been implicated.

Clinical features: a watery diarrhea (4.19) lasting about 3 days, winter dysentery causes a sporadic problem in adult dairy cattle. Spontaneous recovery usually takes

4.19. Winter dysentery in cow: watery feces (Jersey)

place after a few days. Some animals show profuse intestinal hemorrhage, passing large quantities of fresh blood in feces (4.20), and suffer a severe production drop, though deaths are rare. Seroconversion to coronavirus can be used for diagnosis, although many animals in a herd are already seropositive.

Repeated outbreaks are possibly due to the presence of carrier animals.

Differential diagnosis: Johne's disease (4.16), rumenitis or overeating (4.56), BVD, salmonellosis, bovine influenza A (diarrhea with respiratory signs), PPH (9.39).

Management: fresh water and palatable feed should be available. The value of intestinal astringents and protectants is disputed. No vaccine is available.

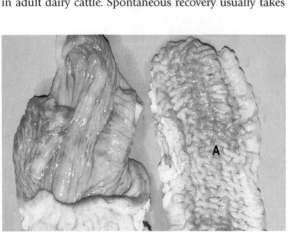

4.18. Johne's disease : normal and abnormal ileum (right) with prominent rugae

4.20. Winter dysentery: specimen showing fresh blood in feces

Gastrointestinal parasitism

The major gastrointestinal parasites of cattle are the stomach (abomasal) worms *Haemonchus placei* (barber's pole worm or large stomach worm, 3–18 mm long male), *Ostertagia ostertagi* (medium or brown stomach worm, 6–9 mm long), and *Trichostrongylus axei* (small stomach worm, 5 mm long). In tropical regions, other species, e.g., *Mecistocirrus digitatus* (up to 4 mm long), are significant. Severe infestations of *Haemonchus* can cause marked anemia, while the major effect of *Ostertagia* and *Trichostrongylus* is a severe, protein-losing gastroenteropathy, characterized by a profuse, watery diarrhea. All three species have the facility for their embryonated eggs or infective larvae to survive in feces for weeks or months at lower temperatures (e.g., over winter) or in drought conditions, until a favorable environment returns.

Of the three species, *Ostertagia ostertagi* is overall the most pathogenic and economically important in most temperate regions of the world, including the UK and much of the USA. As with most gastrointestinal parasites, the most severe effects are seen in growing animals. Nevertheless, it can be a devastatingly debilitating disease in susceptible adults.

Ostertagiasis

Clinical features: cattle are most commonly affected with a chronic, persistent diarrhea and weight loss during their first season at pasture. Type I disease caused by *Ostertagia ostertagi* results from the ingestion of large numbers of L_3 larvae from herbage, starting 3–6 weeks before the onset of clinical signs. Small nodules that are 1–2 mm in diameter are present on and between the abomasal folds on the mucosal surface (4.21). In severe cases a "Morocco leather" or "cobblestone" appearance is evident (4.22). Higher magnification of a severe case shows the thickened rugae (ridges) and the white worms (4.23). Marked edema of the gastrointestinal wall is often present. Type II disease occurs when larvae ingested in the autumn lie dormant in the abomasal glands (as L_4), and then emerge en masse in late winter or early spring to produce a profuse scour and weight loss in housed

4.22. Ostertagiasis with "Morocco leather" appearance of abomasal mucosa

4.23. Ostertagiasis showing thickened abomasal rugae and many white worms

cattle. Note the weight loss, chronic diarrhea, and tenesmus in an older Charolais heifer (4.24).

Oesophagostomum infection

Clinical features: clinical signs tend to be much less severe than with *Ostertagia*. Heavy worm burdens in

4.21. Ostertagiasis with multiple abomasal nodules

4.24. Ostertagiasis type II: chronic stage in wasted heifer showing tenesmus (Charolais)

4.25. *Oesophagostomum* infection: numerous caseated and calcified nodules on distal intestinal serosa (USA)

4.26. Temporary incisors being replaced by permanent teeth

4.27. Grossly excessive wear of incisors, worn down to stumps

calves cause anorexia, severe, dark diarrhea, and weight loss. In older animals the nodules affect gut motility. These nodules may be palpated per rectum. The worms measure 12–15 mm and the head is angled to the body.

4.25 shows the serosal surface of the distal small intestine. Numerous caseated and calcified nodules indicate the presence of *Oesophagostomum radiatum* (nodular worm 12–15 mm long) in an older, resistant animal.

Management of *Ostertagiasis* and *Oesophagostomum* infection: in a clinical outbreak, all animals in the group should be treated with an appropriate broad-spectrum anthelmintic. The group should be moved to a "clean" pasture, and adequate nutrition should be ensured. Strategic management techniques have been developed as preventative measures, varying with worm types, climate, management systems, and economic considerations. In the UK the most common control is anthelmintic therapy of first-season calves from turn-out to late June, by which time all over-wintered larvae will have died.

Dental problems

Clinical features: dental problems are not a common cause of clinical disease in cattle. Occasionally, when the temporary incisors are being replaced by the permanent dentition, 2–3-year-old heifers show difficulty in prehension (4.26) leading to excessive salivation and weight loss. Diets such as heavily impacted self-feed silage leading to excessive incisor wear (4.27) may cause progressive weight loss. The crowns have almost disappeared, resulting in impairment of the animal's foraging ability. Shedding teeth (4.28) can lead to temporary dysphagia and impaired weight gain.

Management: heifers should ideally be milked as a separate group during their first lactation and be given easy-access feed.

Fluorosis

Fluorosis (4.29) leads to mottling and excessive wear of temporary teeth during their development. The more severe fluorine-induced discoloration (4.30) should be differentiated from the staining caused by ingestion of some forms of grass silage. Other signs of fluorosis are seen in 13.31 and 13.32.

Irregular molar wear

Irregular molar wear can sometimes cause masticatory problems. When eating or ruminating, this 8-year-old

4.28. Shedding incisors

4.29. Fluorosis with mottling of temporary teeth (USA)

4.30. Severe fluorosis-induced discoloration of teeth (USA)

bull (4.31) occasionally kept the jaws apart as a result of "locking" the overgrown lingual edge of the upper molars and premolars against the buccal edge of the mandibular cheek teeth. The length of the bilaterally symmetrical overgrowth was about 1 cm. 4.31 shows the typical open "locked" position.

Mandibular fracture

Clinical features: mandibular fractures can occur in calves being kicked by cows or occasionally from iatrogenic trauma, e.g., from farm machinery. In the mature Friesian cow (4.32) with the symphysial fracture, the central incisor was displaced. There was little separation of the two halves of the mandible. A considerable quantity of saliva is being lost. In this case the cause

4.31. Locked jaw position (chronic, intermittent) in bull (Charolais, 8 years old)

4.32. Symphysial fracture in cow, which recovered without surgery (Friesian)

was unknown, and full recovery occurred without treatment.

Management: a recent mandibular symphysial fracture may be stabilized by figure-of-eight wiring or use of a resin block across the incisor teeth. Milk-fed calves commonly continue to suckle and recover without treatment.

Discrete swellings of the head

Actinobacillosis, actinomycosis, and local abscessation related to *Arcanobacterium pyogenes* can present similar clinical features in some cattle. Typically, however, actinobacillosis affects the soft tissues, especially the tongue, while actinomycosis involves bone. Abscessation related to tooth root infection is rare in cattle. A curious disorder or vice of habitual tongue playing, not involving any oral pathology, is shown in 4.33. This Guernsey cow lost a considerable volume of saliva through drooling.

Actinobacillosis ("wooden tongue")

Clinical features: *Actinobacillus lignieresii* preferentially colonizes the soft tissues of the head, especially the tongue. External swelling beneath the jaw may be seen (4.34). It typically causes a localized, firm swelling of the dorsum (D), as in this dairy cow (4.35) and firm, easily palpable, subepithelial masses elsewhere. Actinobacillosis with severe swelling of the tongue may result in its chronic protrusion (4.36). Other parts of the head, such as the nares or facial skin, are sometimes alone affected. Infection may pass down the esophagus, and lesions in the esophageal groove typically cause vomiting of rumen contents or bloat. Other areas of the body (e.g., the limbs (4.37) face and head (4.38), or flanks) may develop cutaneous actinobacillosis. Skin infection usually follows trauma and exposure to a concentrated infective dose of organisms, which are part of the normal flora of the upper GI tract. Such massive lesions are particularly liable to bleed and ulcerate. Most cases tend to occur in mature cattle of dairy breeds.

4

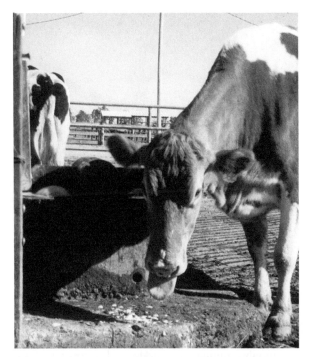

4.33. Habitual tongue-playing in cow. Note saliva on ground (Guernsey)

4.34. Actinobacillosis with severe submandibular swelling

4.35. Actinobacillosis in thickened dorsum of tongue (D)

4.36. Actinobacillosis causing tongue protrusion in cow (Highland)

Differential diagnosis: tooth abscess, actinomycosis, foot-and-mouth disease, snakebite (4.39, showing thickening and ulceration 4 days later).

Management: systemic antibiotics are effective, but prolonged therapy (7–10 days) may be needed. Provide clean feed and water, and avoid access to muddy streams.

4.37. Actinobacillosis of several limbs in Angus steer (Canada)

4.38. Actinobacillosis on mandible

Actinomycosis ("lumpy jaw")

Clinical features: actinomycosis (*Actinomyces bovis*) causes a rarefying periostitis of the maxilla and the mandible, with a surrounding soft-tissue reaction. The Guernsey cow in 4.40 has a right maxillary swelling, and several granulomatous masses have typically broken through the skin. The cow experienced no apparent interference with mastication for 18 months after the swelling was first seen. The crossbred Hereford cow with "lumpy jaw" (4.41) had moderate difficulty in chewing. A large, fist-sized, proliferating mass lies over the angle of the mandible. Any discharge tends to be honey-like, containing hard yellow-white granules ("sulfur granules"). Despite secondary infection, body condition remained good. Dysphagia is usually due to malalignment of molar teeth. A lateral radiograph (4.42) of a 2-year-old heifer with mandibular actinomycosis (in considerable discomfort and rapidly losing weight) shows massive periosteal new bone formation (A) and cavitation (B).

4.40. Actinomycosis with several granulomata on maxillary region of cow (Guernsey)

4.41. Actinomycosis with large granulomatous mass on jaw of cow (Hereford cross)

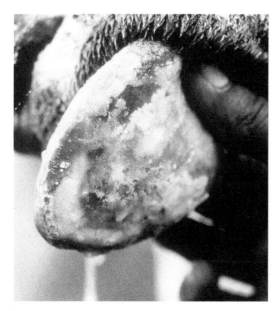

4.39. Snake bite causing severe slough of ventral surface of tongue epithelium

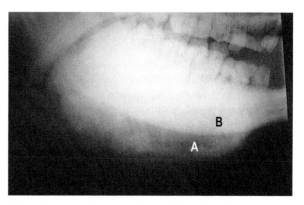

4.42. Lateral radiograph of mandible with actinomycosis showing bone destruction and proliferation

4

4.43. Ameloblastoma proliferating from mandible in heifer (Saler, 11 weeks old)

Differential diagnosis: mandibular abscess (4.48), actinobacillosis (4.34–4.38).

Management: actinomycosis has a poor prognosis despite attempts at debridement and prolonged (7+ days) systemic use of β-lactam antimicrobial drugs (e.g., synthetic penicillins and cephalosporins).

Ameloblastoma

Definition: locally invasive and highly destructive tumor of the jaw.

Clinical features: an 11-week-old Saler heifer presents a mass (4.43) firmly attached to the mandible, which is distorted making prehension very difficult. Euthanasia as surgical removal was impossible. Such soft tissue malignancies are rare.

Differential diagnosis: actinomycosis (4.41), actinobacillosis (4.38).

Malignant edema (necrotic cellulitis)

Etiology: malignant edema is caused by *Clostridium septicum* and results from contaminated wounds in any superficial part of the body, although the head and neck are most commonly affected.

Clinical features: anorexia, pyrexia, and toxemia develop rapidly along with local lesions. In this cow (4.44), infection entered the masseter area of the right cheek to cause a rapidly enlarging and unilateral soft tissue swelling, especially obvious around the right nostril. There was pronounced salivation. The brisket was enlarged with edematous fluid (4.45). Despite prompt, prolonged antibiotic therapy, infection spread to the forelegs and, as in many cases, was fatal. Gas formation is rare.

Differential diagnosis: cutaneous urticaria (blaine) (3.1), abscessation (4.48).

4.44. Malignant edema in right masseteric region of cow (Holstein)

Management: prolonged and aggressive parenteral penicillin plus NSAIDs may cure some early cases. Some benefit from drainage of foci. Although clostridial vaccines are available, most cases are sporadic and herd vaccination is rarely indicated.

Alveolar periostitis (Cara inchada, "swollen face")

Definition: severe periodontal disease associated with secondary bacterial infection in young cattle of unknown etiology.

Clinical features: alveolar periostitis is a major problem in some parts of South America, such as Brazil. Periodontal disease affects the sockets of the upper

4.45. Malignant edema with massive enlargement of brisket in cow (Holstein)

4.46. Alveolar periostitis (cara inchada): specimen with tooth loss and maxillary changes in steer (Zebu) (Brazil)

premolars and molars in calves following a severe gingivitis and secondary bacterial infection (*Arcanobacterium pyogenes* and *Prevotella melaninogenica*). The first sign is uni- or bilateral swelling of the cheek as a result of impaction by pasture grass. Autopsy examination reveals loss or marked displacement of several temporary teeth, particularly premolars two and three, and a massive periosteal and osteolytic reaction in the related maxilla (4.46, 4.47). On pastures of guinea grass (*Panicum maximum*), which causes traumatic damage to the gingiva, the condition leads to malnutrition and sometimes death. The 18-month-old mixed Zebu steer from the Mato Grosso (4.46) has lost the right second and third upper premolars (A) and the left second premolar (B). Loss of the surrounding cement has led to deep pockets on the labial side of the right arcade (C). The steer was severely emaciated. 4.47 shows a similar type of animal. A striking, chronic, ossifying periostitis affects the region around the roots of P2 and P3, explaining the likelihood of tooth loss.

Submandibular abscess

Clinical features: caused by *Arcanobacterium pyogenes*, a smooth and localized soft-tissue swelling, discharging pus, lies over the horizontal ramus of the left mandible (4.48). It developed rapidly over 3 weeks and resolved slowly.

Differential diagnosis: actinomycosis (4.40), actinobacillosis (4.34), fracture of the mandible (4.32).

4.47. Alveolar periostitis: bone specimen with severe periostitis (Brazil)

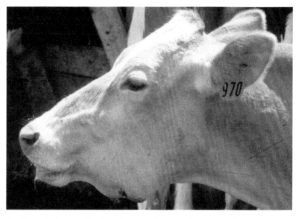

4.48. Submandibular abscess in cow (Guernsey)

Management: surgical drainage and flushing. Systemic antibiotics may be unnecessary.

Pharyngeal and retropharyngeal swelling

Pharyngeal and retropharyngeal swellings can range from being innocuous to rapidly fatal. Careful external and oral/pharyngeal examination is essential. A swelling may be indicative of systemic disease elsewhere, such as right heart failure manifested as submandibular and retropharyngeal edema (6.2). The swelling may involve retropharyngeal and parotid lymph nodes in a neoplastic reaction (12.74). Severe reactions in the submucosal tissues of the pharynx, with potentially dire consequences to the airway and possibly death, can result from ingestion of neat caustic soda (sodium hydroxide) from improperly mixed caustic wheat, or anthelmintic bolus gun injuries. The introduction of a small amount of irritant material (e.g., poloxalene for bloat control) through an accidental puncture wound, or other forms of extensive lacerations to the pharyngeal wall, cause severe edema, cellulitis, and pose a major problem (see below).

Drenching gun injury

Clinical features: perforation of the pharyngeal wall by a drenching gun caused a septic cellulitis leading to the grossly enlarged submandibular and parotid regions (4.49). One consequence of this cellulitis was a malodorous, purulent nasal and oral discharge. The steer was pyrexic and anorexic. Autopsy examination of another case (4.50) revealed masses of inspissated pus beneath the pharyngeal and laryngeal mucosae, which had caused respiratory embarrassment (inspiratory stridor). Note the congestion of the mucosal surface of the epiglottis.

Incorrect dosing techniques can result in anthelmintic boluses penetrating the pharyngeal mucosa, migrating down the neck, and producing severe respiratory distress due to foreign body reaction and airway obstruction.

4

4

4.49.   Septic cellulitis following drenching gun injury in (Angus) steer

Management: aggressive and prolonged antibiotics and anti-inflammatories are needed, but effective therapy is very difficult in severe cases with extensive septic cellulitis. Respiratory obstruction is possible (emergency tracheotomy) or rumen tympany (trocarization), but most cases fail to respond and culling is the usual economic option.

Retropharyngeal abscess

Clinical features: a discrete and relatively painless fluctuating, tennis ball-sized mass lies in the retropharyngeal region (4.51). The spread of infection (compare 4.49) was limited by the development of a fibrous capsule. Abscessation in this region is commonly caused by ingestion of sticks and thorns, although it may be the result of accidental pharyngeal damage from drenching or balling guns, probangs, or other rigid instruments (see above).

4.50.   Drenching gun injury (autopsy) with massive septic pharyngeal cellulitis (USA)

4.51.   Discrete retropharyngeal abscess

Management: most abscesses eventually develop superficial softer areas for drainage, though deep-seated abscesses can be hazardous due to the proximity of other structures, e.g., carotid artery, jugular vein, or parotid salivary gland.

Esophageal disorders

Esophageal obstruction (choke)

Clinical features: a potato is lodged two-thirds of the way down the cervical esophagus to the left of the hand (4.52). The animal was uncomfortable and drooling as a result of its inability to swallow saliva. Since eructation was impeded, it also had rumen tympany. Common sites of esophageal obstruction are just dorsal to the larynx and at the thoracic inlet. In cattle, esophageal foreign bodies tend to be solid objects, such as apples, large portions of turnips or beets, or corncobs (maize). Other suspicious signs of esophageal obstruction include extension of the head and neck, dyspnea, occasional coughing, and chewing movements. A cervical esophageal foreign body is readily palpated externally.

Differential diagnosis: acute rumenitis (4.56–4.60), traumatic reticulitis, oral lesions, rabies (9.33–9.35).

4.52.   Esophageal obstruction by potato in heifer

4.53. Chronic megaesophagus in heifer (Charolais, 15 months old)

4.54. Cud regurgitated in mild rumen acidosis (SARA)

Management: some foreign bodies can be pushed towards the pharynx by external manipulation and, using a gag, removed manually. Any severe ruminal tympany should be promptly relieved by trocarization. Other conservative therapy (spasmolytics, e.g., acepromazine, or sedative and muscle relaxants, e.g., xylazine) is preferable to hazardous attempts to push the object downwards with a probang.

Megaesophagus

Definition: chronic dilatation and atony of the esophagus.

Clinical features: the entire cervical esophagus (4.53) is grossly distended (about 5–6 cm in diameter). Contrast radiography revealed a similar distension of most of the thoracic esophagus. The abnormality had been first observed at 1 year of age. Clinical signs included frequent regurgitation. The 15-month-old Charolais heifer was observed for 1 year and almost completely recovered. Megaesophagus is rare and, although usually congenital, this case was probably secondary to a systemic infection.

Differential diagnosis: esophageal obstruction.

Management: diet.

Rumen and reticulum

Rumen acidosis (rumenitis)

Definition: ruminal inflammation resulting from excessively rapid fermentation following overeating of grain (corn), or other high-starch/low-fiber diets. SARA (subacute ruminal acidosis) is an increasing problem in high-yielding dairy herds.

Clinical features: low-grade rumen acidosis can present clinically as rumen atony, cud regurgitation (4.54) and a matted sweaty coat. Passage of loose yellow feces as in this animal (4.55) leads to extensive soiling of

the tail and hindquarters. Tail swishing often produces fecal soiling along the back. More severe overeating can result in rapid carbohydrate fermentation, severe rumenitis, metabolic acidosis, and a subsequent laminitis (7.72). Affected cattle are very dull, weak, ataxic, or recumbent. A light-colored diarrhea containing grain particles may be seen (4.56). Ruminal pH is usually very acidic (pH < 5.5). 4.57 shows areas of sloughed ruminal epithelium and intense serosal hemorrhage in a 10-month-old Simmental bull which died 24 hours after unlimited access to fodder beet. Whole fragments of undigested fodder beet are clearly visible (A). Four to six days after a grain overload, mycotic or fusobacterial rumenitis may be seen (4.58), comprising sharply defined, thick oval ulcers that

4.55. Rumen acidosis with loose yellow feces

4.56. Rumen acidosis with severe yellowish diarrhea

4

4.57. Fatal rumen acidosis with (pink) sloughed ruminal epithelium (autopsy) in bull (Simmental, 10 months old)

4.58. Mycotic or fusobacterial rumenitis (autopsy) (USA)

are often red or dark. A close-up view of a more chronic rumenitis (4.59) shows a rumen fold separating the disorganized and necrotic rumenal papillae (A) from more normal papillae (B). In rumenitis colonized by *Fusobacteria* and fungi, healing eventually occurs after sloughing of the necrotic layers, contraction of the ulcer, and peripheral epithelial regeneration, resulting in stellate scar formation. The rumen is then left with a reduced absorptive capacity, and possible secondary hepatic abscessation.

The omasum in 4.60 shows a fungal infection (most likely due to *Aspergillus* species) following the accidental

4.59. Chronic rumen acidosis showing necrotic rumen papillae (A) at autopsy

4.60. Omasitis due to fungal infection (USA)

ingestion of moldy feed, e.g., cereals or beans. Changes are most common in the ruminoreticulum (4.58) and omasal involvement is rare.

Differential diagnosis: winter dysentery, bloat, and diarrhea from other causes, e.g., sudden feed change.

Management: cases of mild acidosis will resolve without treatment. More severe cases require oral antibiotics (to reduce rumen fermentation), NSAIDs (to suppress laminitis), and antacids and B vitamins (since ruminal vitamin B synthesis is depressed by acidosis). Advanced cases with a metabolic acidosis benefit from i.v. sodium bicarbonate infusion and even evacuation of rumen contents (rumenotomy or esophageal flushing).

Prevention is based on dietary management. Cattle on ad-lib cereals should always have access to palatable fiber (e.g., straw) and never be allowed to be hungry. High-yielding dairy cows need adequate digestible and long fiber to balance a high-starch diet. Ideal concentrate:fiber ratio should never exceed 60:40.

Rumen tympany ("bloat")

Definition: accumulation of gas in a distended rumen. The gas may be free or present as a foam. (See also bloat in younger calves, 2.38.)

Clinical features: the Holstein heifer in 4.61 has an obvious distension of the left paralumbar fossa. The swelling may extend above the level of the lumbar spine, as seen in the Hereford steer (4.62). Both animals had a gaseous as opposed to a foamy (or frothy) bloat. Extreme cases may die from increased intra-abdominal pressure leading to cardiac and respiratory failure, often with inhalation of rumen contents.

Differential diagnosis: distinguish gas bloat from frothy bloat; esophageal obstruction (4.52), an esophageal groove mass (4.63), traumatic reticulitis (4.67), rumenal atony. (For bloat in a calf, see 2.38.)

Management: frothy bloat responds well to oral surfactants such as paloxalene. Gas bloat can usually be

4.61. Rumen tympany ("bloat") in heifer (Holstein)

4.64. Posture of heifer in abdominal pain with legs extended and head to flank (Holstein) (USA)

4.62. Severe rumen tympany in steer (Hereford)

relieved by stomach tube, but extreme cases require trocarization. Prevention depends on avoidance of causative agents.

Ruminal neoplasia

Clinical features: this pedunculated mass (4.63) is a benign papilloma. Lying at the proximal end of the esophageal groove, it caused partial obstruction of the lower esophageal sphincter, resulting in an intermittent

4.63. Ruminal papilloma (autopsy) which caused intermittent bloat

ruminal tympany. Esophageal groove obstructions often also lead to vomiting.

Differential diagnosis: exploratory rumenotomy may be needed to differentiate benign or malignant (squamous cell carcinoma (SCC)) neoplasia from actinobacillosis of the esophageal groove, chronic reticuloperitonitis or reticular wall abscessation. (See 4.67 for another ruminoreticular neoplasm (fibroma).)

Abdominal pain

In comparison with the horse, such signs of pain as seen in this heifer (4.64) are uncommon. The forefeet are placed further forward than normal, presumably in an attempt to reduce tension on the abdominal viscera. The head is turned towards the flank. The tail is slightly elevated (indicative of tenesmus) and the heifer is kicking at the belly with a hind foot. The stance suggests an intestinal problem. Posterior abdominal pain can result in tenesmus that may not necessarily reflect an alimentary origin, e.g., babesiosis (12.39–12.43), cystitis (10.14), or urethritis.

Traumatic reticulitis (reticuloperitonitis, "tire wire disease")

Definition: perforation of reticular wall and parietal peritoneum (usually diaphragm) with development of localized or generalized peritonitis.

Clinical features: Cattle with acute reticuloperitonitis are pyrexic, slightly bloated, and typically grunt during reticular movements unless there is ruminoreticular stasis. Affected cattle may rapidly become dehydrated, one sign of which is obvious skin "tenting" (4.65): the skin fold remains for 3–10 seconds or more (indicating approximately 6–12% dehydration). They appear dejected, have an arched back, raised tail, sunken eyes as a result of the dehydration, weight loss, and an empty flank and "tucked up" belly due to lack of rumen fill (4.66). They are often reluctant to move due to abdominal pain.

4

4.65.   Skin tenting indicative of dehydration (10%)

4.66.   "Tucked up" belly resulting from poor rumen fill

This section (4.67) of the reticular wall illustrates the typical wires that may perforate the wall to cause a localized or generalized peritonitis (4.90, 4.91), hepatic abscessation (4.100), or may travel cranially to produce a septic pericarditis (6.5). An incidental abnormality in

4.67.   Reticular wall (autopsy) with several typical wires (foreign bodies) (USA)

4.68.   Cardiac tamponade and tire wire (↗). Pericardiac sac filled with frank blood-note wire

this reticulum (4.67) was a discrete pedunculated fibroma (A). Wires contained within fragmenting car tires, originally used to keep grass silage sheets in place or left in a field corner, are a frequent source. An autopsy case (4.68) shows cardiac tamponade due to a tire wire which having perforated initially the diaphragm, has traveled through the epicardium into the myocardium, rupturing a major vessel which has pumped blood into the pericardial sac, resulting a sudden interference with cardiac activity. Herd outbreaks may arise when an entire tire is accidentally chopped up in the feed wagon.

Differential diagnosis: left (4.76) or right (4.78) displaced abomasum, abomasal ulceration with perforation (4.72), cecal dilatation (4.89), bacterial endocarditis (6.3), rumen acidosis (4.58, 4.59), other digestive upsets.

Management: prognosis is good in early acute cases following rumenotomy and removal of penetrating wire in reticulum. Alternative medical management involves antibacterials for several days, elevation of the forequarters, and oral administration of a magnet which is useful both for prophylaxis and treatment. Prognosis is hopeless when penetrating wire has perforated the pericardium (traumatic pericarditis, 6.6) or myocardium leading to cardiac tamponade (4.68)

4.69. Vagal indigestion (Hoflund syndrome) with severe distension from excessive rumen fluid (Netherlands)

Abomasum

Abomasal obstructive syndrome (vagal indigestion, "Hoflund syndrome")

Definition: the cause of vagal indigestion, or Hoflund syndrome, is a functional disturbance of the normal motility of the forestomachs or the abomasum, or of all compartments.

Clinical features: the silhouette of the abdominal wall shows a massive, left-sided swelling due to an accumulation of fluid, primarily in the ruminoreticulum (4.69). After pumping out 90 liters, the flanks became almost symmetrical (4.70). The distension is characteristically in the upper left and lower right flanks, resulting in the so-called "ten-to-four" appearance. 4.71 is a typical example.

Ruminoreticular distension that results from vagal dysfunction due to chronic reticuloperitonitis is the most common manifestation. Severe ruminal distension is most marked in the left sublumbar fossa and low down in the right flank (so-called "papple-shaped", i.e., pear × apple).

4.70. Same cow as in 4.69 after removal of 90 liters of fluid from rumen (Netherlands)

4.71. Vagal indigestion: typical dorsal left flank, ventral right flank distension (USA)

Discrete omasal obstruction (as opposed to secondary abomasal obstruction) due to reticuloperitonitis is rare. When compared with 4.69, the abdominal silhouette of the 2-year-old Holstein bull in 4.71 is similarly asymmetrical, showing distension of the upper left (ruminoreticulum) and lower right (omasum, and to a lesser extent ruminoreticulum) flanks. The cause of the omasal obstruction was secondary impaction due to a reticular wall abscess (foreign body: wire) and a localized reticuloperitonitis. Mechanical causes, such as neoplastic infiltration near the pylorus, can lead to similar effects. Diagnosis depends on exploratory laparotomy.

Differential diagnosis: chronic traumatic reticulitis, peritonitis, rumen tympany, abomasal impaction, obstruction of the reticulo-omasal orifice.

Management: diagnosis of the specific cause involves an exploratory laparotomy and rumenotomy. Evacuation of rumen contents may improve motility temporarily. Symptomatic treatment is necessary. The prognosis is often poor.

Abomasal ulceration

Clinical features: abomasal ulceration occurs in mature dairy and beef cattle and in calves (2.27–2.29). Some cases in adults are the result of primary diseases such as infiltrative lymphosarcoma, and systemic infections such as BVD and malignant bovine catarrh. In high-yielding dairy cows, although the cause is unknown, ulcers are usually associated with stress and high-concentrate rations. Multiple abomasal ulcers may occur in calves (2.28). There are four types of ulcer. Type I causes no clinically apparent disease and is common. Type II is a bleeding ulcer that, if persistent, results in progressive anemia. Types III and IV cause an acute localized or generalized peritonitis with signs of pain, and Type IV is almost always fatal. Animals are dull, with a drop in yield, often a subnormal temperature, and general signs of anemia.

The Guernsey cow in 4.72 had abdominal pain due to a Type III (perforating) abomasal ulcer causing a

4

4.72. Abomasal ulceration: passing of dark tarry feces by cow (Guernsey)

4.74. Healing abomasal ulcers (autopsy)

localized peritonitis. She passed black, tarry feces containing much digested blood (4.72). Cows sometimes die following severe blood loss into the abomasal lumen. Autopsy examination (4.73) reveals numerous ulcers, several filled with blood (A), and a diffuse abomasitis. The pathology is similar to that of the calfhood disease (2.27–2.29), with localized or generalized peritonitis as possible sequelae. Healing abomasal ulcers (4.74) show scar tissue causing contraction of the abomasal wall in a stellate pattern. Some bleeding was still occurring.

Differential diagnosis: traumatic reticulitis, abomasitis, abomasal lymphoma (lymphosarcoma) (4.75), jejunal hemorrhagic syndrome (4.83–4.85).

Management: depending on the symptomatology, broad-spectrum antibiotics are indicated in perforating ulcers, whilst fluid therapy including blood may be given to dehydrated animals and cases of bleeding ulcers. Unfortunately fluids increase blood pressure and in many cases will precipitate further hemorrhage from the ulcer.

Abomasal lymphoma (lymphosarcoma)

Etiology and pathogenesis: adult lymphosarcoma is caused by the bovine leukosis virus (BLV). The tumor incidence varies widely. Enzootic leukosis affects mature cattle, and other structures commonly affected include lymph nodes, heart, and retrobulbar tissue (8.42).

This specimen from an old Holstein cow shows thickened and irregular abomasal rugae as a result of lymphoma infiltration (4.75). Neoplastic infiltration was widespread. The discrete, dark, punched-out areas are ulcers, indicating that the two conditions can occur together.

Management: diagnosis ultimately requires histological confirmation. Control in a herd is difficult but regular serology may facilitate removal of positive carriers. (See also 12.74–12.81.)

Abomasal surgical conditions

In areas of intensive management, left and to a lesser extent right abomasal displacements are common

4.73. Abomasal ulceration (A) and hemorrhage in cow (autopsy) (Guernsey)

4.75. Abomasal lymphoma infiltrating rugae (autopsy)

conditions in dairy cattle. Right abomasal torsion can be a serious secondary complication of right abomasal displacement. Most cases of mechanical displacement of this type occur in high-yielding cows in early lactation, and are preceded by a period of ruminal and abomasal atony. Many cows will have had periparturient problems such as retained placenta, ketosis, metritis, mastitis, for dietary-induced rumen acidosis (SARA) in the preceding weeks.

Left displaced abomasum (LDA)

Clinical features: the displaced abomasum is situated almost entirely beneath the rib cage on the left, where it can be detected by percussion and auscultation. The caudal, dorsal portion may extend behind the last rib to form a palpable, soft swelling which may on rectal examination be distinguished from the underlying rumen in the paralumbar fossa. In 4.76 the abomasum (A) may be seen through a left paralumbar vertical incision lying between the cranial edge of the incision and the spleen (B), which is cranial to the visible portion (C) of the rumen wall. LDA presents with variable clinical signs, often a sudden loss of appetite for concentrates and precipitous drop in yield. Other cows have moderate inappetance, weight loss, and a secondary ketosis. With this slow loss of condition due to partial inappetance, the bulge (A) of the abomasum may then become more obvious in the left flank (4.77).

Differential diagnosis: right displaced abomasum (4.78), cecal torsion (4.88), primary ketosis.

Management: conservative correction by rolling, confinement to a loose box, and a high roughage intake can cure up to 30% of cases. Surgical abomasopexy by one of several techniques, or a "toggling" procedure are preferred, and the prognosis is then good.

Right displaced abomasum (RDA)

Clinical features: clinical signs are similar to left displacement, but a tympanitic abomasum is detectable by

4.77. LDA with bulge in left flank (A) of cow (Guernsey)

percussion on the right side. In this Guernsey cow (4.78) the distended abomasum is seen through a vertical right flank paralumbar incision about 7 cm caudal to the last rib. The remainder of the abomasum is located medial to the costal arch. The greater omentum containing the descending duodenum (A) is seen caudal to the abomasal swelling (B).

Differential diagnosis: left displaced abomasum, abomasal, intestinal or cecal torsion, ketosis, abomasal ulceration.

Management: mild cases of RDA may slowly respond to medical therapy (meclofenamic acid, spasmolytics) and dietary management. More advanced cases require surgical drainage and abomasopexy. After removal of the large volumes of gas and fluid, most cases will recover slowly.

4.78. Right displaced abomasum (RDA): (A) descending duodenum visible caudal to abomasum (B) through flank incision in cow (Guernsey)

4.76. Left displaced abomasum (LDA) (A), seen through left flank incision in cow (Friesian)

4.79. Abomasal torsion at autopsy showing (A) abomasum, (B) ruminoreticulum, and (C) duodenum

4.80. Cow with abomasal impaction (Holstein, Germany)

Abomasal torsion

Clinical features: abomasal torsion with dilatation is clinically severe, and affected cows are dull, sometimes recumbent, totally anorexic, dehydrated, in shock and have an empty rectum. The dilated abomasum can be percussed on the right flank and may be palpable per rectum. An autopsy specimen (4.79) of the abomasum (A), ruminoreticulum (B) and duodenum (C) shows a complex torsion of both the abomasum and omasum. Typically, the cow was found in extreme shock. The abomasal fluid volume exceeded 90 liters (normal volume: 10–20 liters).

Management: most cases should be culled. Any attempt at treatment involves correction of the fluid imbalance and right-sided abomasal drainage followed by attempted reposition of the abomasum.

Abomasal impaction

Clinical features: herd outbreaks usually result from consumption of large quantities of poor-quality roughage in cold weather by young beef cows (e.g., Canadian prairies, Saskatchewan). Sporadic isolated cases are seen in dairy cows secondary to vagal indigestion (p. 71). Signs include anorexia, reduced feces, and increasing distension of both flanks ("10-to-4" appearance). A 5-year-old Holstein cow, fed maize silage and grass silage (4.80), presented with a massive, firm abdominal distension. At autopsy (4.81) the abomasal volume was 60–70 liters, and included 15–20 kg sand. The abomasal mucosa was very congested and, after emptying, some sand is still evident between the folds. This was the only cow affected within the herd, suggesting the impaction could have been related to a pre-existing vagal indigestion.

Differential diagnosis: vagal indigestion (4.69–4.71), omasal impaction, intestinal obstruction (lipomatosis, 4.101), diffuse peritonitis (4.90). (See also 4.82 for trichobezoar.)

Management: salvage slaughter; avoid impaction by adequate good-quality roughage, when available.

Abomasal trichobezoar

Definition: rounded mass of felted hair and plant material distending and partially obstructing abomasum.

Clinical features: seen in younger cattle (e.g. 6–12 months) in certain regions and under specific husbandry conditions trichobezoars (4.82) are comparatively rare in cattle. Signs are nonspecific with inappetance and weight loss, but ballottement in calves can be diagnostic. Frequently an abomasal trichobezoar also causes a secondary abomasitis and associated ulceration.

Management: surgery on individual valuable animals, dietary change, and husbandry management, e.g., treatment for lice to reduce the frequency of licking the haircoat.

4.81. Cow of 4.80 showing severe abomasal mucosal hyperemia and remains of massive sand accumulation (Germany)

4.82. Trichobezoar in abomasum of calf at surgery (Chianina) (Italy)

Small intestine

Jejunal hemorrhagic syndrome (JHS), hemorrhagic bowel syndrome (HBS), hemorrhagic gut syndrome (HGS), "hemorrhagic enteritis"

Definition: a relatively recently described acute condition of milking dairy cows, usually fatal, of unknown etiology, but associated with high yields and high feed intakes.

Clinical features: possibly fleeting signs suggestive of clinical ketosis (recumbent cow unwilling to go to milking parlor). Most cases have sudden onset (4.83) of shock, total inappetance, and severe anemia. Distension of right flank and ballottement reveal extensive fluid-filled intestinal loops ventrally, and gas in paralumbar fossa and beneath rib cage. In cases surviving more than

4.84. Jejunal hemorrhagic syndrome (JHS): right flank standing laparotomy showing typical loop of grossly distended, blood-filled jejunum (Holstein, USA)

12 hours profuse dark, tarry feces may be passed, with early recumbency and death within 36 hours. Right flank exploratory laparotomy discloses multiple jejunal loops distended with bloody fluid (4.84). Autopsy reveals massive whole blood clots in numerous jejunal loops (4.85) and petechiae on the intestinal serosa, as well as early peritonitis (serosal tags evident).

Differential diagnosis: acute abomasal ulceration with perforation and early peritonitis, acute jejunal intussusception, right abomasal torsion.

Management: early recognition of JHS is vital if an attempt is to be made to correct the massive fluid and blood loss. Few peracute cases survive. Improved dietary management is indicated.

4.83. Jejunal hemorrhagic syndrome (JHS): downer cow, Holstein. Note depression, open mouth breathing and raised hackles (hair coat), symptomatic of severe stress, in right paralumbar fossa (USA)

4.85. Jejunal hemorrhagic syndrome (JHS): autopsy with several loops of distended hemorrhagic jejunum, to right of which lie other fluid- and gas-filled loops. Note early fibrin tags indicative of peritonitis (USA)

4

4.86. Jejunal intussusception (B) at exploratory surgery

Jejunal torsion and intussusception ("twisted gut")

Definition: twisting of jejunum on itself and telescoping of small intestinal segment.

Clinical features: intussusception, though sporadic, is the most common cause of small intestinal obstruction in cattle. Occurring at any age, it initially causes severe abdominal pain. Progressive shock develops. The rectum is totally void of feces. In larger cattle torsion may be detectable on rectal examination as a tight mesenteric band passing obliquely across the abdomen. In 4.86 the darker loop of small intestine (A), showing marked congestion and subserosal hemorrhage, particularly on the mesenteric border, is the segment of bowel through which the intussusception has passed. Dilated proximal intestine is seen at B. The point of invagination of the intussusception, which is not visible in this picture, lies tightly knotted deeply below the position of the fingers.

An autopsy case of massive jejunal torsion is seen in (4.87) with most jejunal loops dilated and discolored, as

4.87. Complex intussusception and torsion (autopsy)

4.88. Severe abdominal distension in jejunal obstruction and torsion

is the mesenteric suspension with patchy areas of hemorrhage. The abomasum lies adjacent to these loops. Such cases are usually acute and fatal.

Affected animals often have a grossly distended abdomen (4.88) due to fluid accumulation in the prestenotic small intestinal loops, abomasum, and ruminoreticulum.

Differential diagnosis: abomasal torsion (4.79), jejunal hemorrhagic syndrome (4.83, 4.84).

Management: early cases are sometimes amenable to surgical correction (resection and anastomosis). However, most cases should be promptly culled. Logical preventive measures to reduce the alleged initiating factor for intussusception (intestinal irritation) are parasite control and dietary management.

Large intestine
Cecal dilatation and torsion

Clinical features: affected cows are dull, partially anorexic and have a depressed yield. Onset may be slow and subtle. The dilated cecum can be percussed in the caudal upper right flank and be palpated per rectum (slightly mobile "loaf of bread" shape). Following cecal displacement and distension, the Holstein cow (4.89) developed an acute (painful) abdomen within 48 hours. The enlarged cecum was appreciable on rectal palpation. The cecal apex has been prolapsed through a dorsal and caudal right flank laparotomy incision (4.89), but most of the cecum still lies within the abdominal cavity. The peritoneal surface is slightly congested. Many cases of simple cecal dilatation are asymptomatic. Some develop into cecal torsion and show more severe pain and depression. Others may even recover spontaneously from dilatation.

4.89. Cecal torsion in cow with its apex prolapsed at surgery (Holstein)

4.90. Early generalized peritonitis over greater omentum at autopsy (USA)

Differential diagnosis: right displaced abomasum, ketosis.

Management: many cases respond to spasmolytics and dietary control. Surgical drainage may be needed when viability of the cecal wall should be checked.

Peritonitis

Definition: inflammation of the parietal and visceral peritoneum.

Clinical features: it may be localized or generalized, acute or chronic. It is commonly secondary to contamination of the abdominal cavity, e.g., secondary to traumatic reticulitis or cesarian section. In active disease, guarding of the abdomen results in a stiff gait (see p. 69). The bovine peritoneum and greater omentum have a remarkable facility to wall off leaks of bowel contents and localized areas of abscessation. This process often results in few or no complications in the cranial part of the abdomen. Adhesions developing in the caudal part can cause progressive bowel obstruction. In 4.90 the visceral and parietal peritoneum (rumen, jejunum, and greater omentum) is covered with a fibrinous and purulent exudate, typical of early generalized peritonitis. The changes are more advanced and chronic in another case (4.91), resulting from septic reticuloperitonitis (see also 4.67).

Typical clinical cases of active peritonitis are dull, pyrexic, often partially anorexic and cows have a reduced milk yield. More chronic cases are in poor bodily condition. Rectal examination reveals an empty rumen, and a typical "doughy" feel to attempts to palpate abdominal viscera.

Other common causes of peritonitis are perforated abomasal ulcers, either in calfhood (2.29) or in adult life (4.73), and rupture of the small intestine following uncorrected intussusception or small intestinal torsion.

Neonatal peritonitis may occur following the rupture of a distended small intestine proximal to an atretic bowel (1.22).

Diagnosis: peritonitis may be suspected from the clinical signs and rectal palpation. Abdominal (ventral) paracentesis may yield suspect fluid for cytological and cultural examination.

Management: fluid therapy, aggressive broad-spectrum antimicrobial therapy, NSAIDs. Most cases are best culled.

Ascites

Definition: abnormal accumulation of serous (edematous) fluid in the abdominal cavity.

Clinical features: As with peritonitis, this fluid eventually leads to a pear-shaped silhouette (4.92). Ascitic fluid is serous or edematous in nature and is usually sterile. This old Galloway cow had hepatic cirrhosis resulting

4.91. Advanced chronic peritonitis at autopsy following septic reticuloperitonitis

4

4.92. Ascites showing typical pear-shaped silhouette in aged cow (Galloway)

from chronic severe fascioliasis. Compare intestinal obstruction (4.88). The abdomen is rarely painful on palpation, unlike peritonitis (p. 77). Diagnosis is confirmed by a midline abdominal tap (sterile needle).

Differential diagnosis: peritonitis, (4.90), hydrops amnii, hydrops allantois (10.54), abomasal impaction (4.80).

Management: most cases are incurable and should be culled.

Hepatic diseases

Clinical signs of liver disease are variable and relate to its wide range of functions. These include bile production, synthesis of specific plasma components, detoxification, storage, and a variety of metabolic processes.

Its large functional reserve results in the signs of disease usually becoming evident only when hepatic damage is extensive. There are few characteristic signs of malfunction, and diagnosis often presents a major challenge to the clinician. Several specific diseases of the liver cause reduced weight gain and slaughterhouse condemnation of the liver (abscessation, fluke infestation). Ancillary diagnostic aids include enzyme estimation (sorbitol dehydrogenase (SDH), glutamate dehydrogenase (GDH), γ-glutamyl transferase (GGT)) and percutaneous hepatic biopsy.

Examples of the hepatic diseases illustrated below include fascioliasis resulting from severe parasitism, necrotic hepatitis caused by *Clostridium novyi* type B (*oedematiens*), and hepatic abscessation secondary to rumenitis (*Fusobacterium necrophorum*). Although not specifically involving the liver, other forms of fluke are also included in this section. Fatty liver syndrome produced by ill-defined nutritional and metabolic imbalance is described in Chapter 9 (9.9), and photosensitization secondary to hepatic disease in Chapter 3 (3.3–3.9).

4.93. Liver in severe fascioliasis with massive fibrosis of bile ducts

Fascioliasis (common liver fluke infection)

Definition: disease caused by infestation with *Fasciola*, also termed distomatosis.

Clinical features: an increasing problem in many regions, low-grade fluke infestation produces nonspecific clinical signs such as poor condition, reduced performance (growth and milk yield and quality), and anemia. Autopsy reveals the liver becomes fibrotic with enlargement, the bile ducts grossly thickened, and mature *Fasciola hepatica* flukes occupy the lumen (4.93, 4.94). The walls may eventually become calcified. The

4.94. *Fasciola hepatica* flukes and thickened bile ducts

visceral surface becomes irregular and granular in appearance. The associated fat in ligamentous attachments is lost, leaving little but the grayish peritoneal surface as emaciation develops. Clinical cases become hypoproteinemic, developing ventral and submandibular edema. Ascites (4.92) is a common result. Frequently there is liver condemnation at abattoir.

Diagnosis: in subacute and chronic disease, variable numbers of eggs may be detected in feces. An absence of fluke eggs does not eliminate the presence of fluke. Plasma GGT is elevated in cattle with bile duct damage. Serology will detect antibodies to fluke. Autopsy appearance is diagnostic.

Differential diagnosis: hemonchosis, ostertagiasis.

Management: grazing management and flukicidal drugs. However, some drugs kill only adult flukes, others a wider range of stages of the life cycle. Many are not licensed for use in dairy cattle, so control can be difficult.

Paramphistomiasis (rumen or stomach flukes)

Clinical features: even the relatively large numbers of soft, pink, pear-shaped, adult flukes seen attached to the rumen wall (4.95) cause few or no clinical signs, particularly in older cattle. However, proximally migrating immature worms hatching from metacercarial cysts attached to the duodenum may lead to ulceration and clinical signs including unthriftiness, diarrhea, and death in young animals. Several different species of fluke

including *P. cervi*, *P. microbothrium*, and *P. ichikawai* are involved. Planorbid snails act as intermediate hosts, the life cycle being similar to *Fasciola hepatica*. Paramphistomiasis and fascioliasis may occur together, leading to a more severe syndrome.

Diagnosis and management: see above for fascioliasis. Treat with oxyclozanide for adult paraphistome infections in rumen. Removal of animals from infected pastures, where metacercaria may survive for 2–3 months after pastures have dried out.

Schistosomiasis (blood flukes): Bilharzia

Definition: disease caused by trematode *Schistosoma* spp. with chronic hemorrhagic enteritis, anemia, and emaciation in a group of cattle, many dying after months.

Clinical features: eight species of *Schistosoma* have been reported throughout Africa, the Middle East, and Asia. Cercariae, released into water from the intermediate snail host, penetrate the skin or mucous membranes. 4.96 shows a pair of elongated flukes in a blood vessel of the stretched mesentery (A), with the female lying in a longitudinal groove of the male. Flukes may be up to 30 mm long. Pathogenic species are primarily found in mesenteric blood vessels, although one species, *S. nasale*, inhabits the nasal mucosa. The major clinical signs of hemorrhagic enteritis, anemia, and emaciation are seen when the spiny eggs pass through the gut wall. In the hepatic form, granulomas form around the eggs. Lesions may also be found in the liver, lungs and bladder. *S. nasale* (4.97) produces a proliferative reaction of granulomatous masses, seen in this median section through the nasal turbinate bones. Abscesses rupture to release pus and eggs into the nasal cavity. The effect is chronic nasal obstruction and dyspnea. The parasite inhabits the veins of the mucosa. *S. nasale* is a problem in the Indian subcontinent, Malaysia, and the Caribbean. In the human, cercariae cause "swimmer's itch" and "swamp itch".

4.95. Paramphistomiasis, with adult flukes on rumen wall (South Africa)

4.96. Schistosomiasis: adult flukes in mesenteric vessel (South Africa)

4

4.97. *Schistosoma nasale* in nasal turbinate bones (Belgium)

Diagnosis: history and clinical signs are inadequate for diagnosis. Eggs must be demonstrated in feces, rectal scrapings, or nasal mucus.

Management: in problem regions, e.g., China, where zoonotic spread is widespread, large-scale chemotherapeutic campaigns (e.g., praziquantel), molluskicides, and habitat and management changes are effective in control.

Infectious necrotic hepatitis ("Black disease")

Definition: an acute toxemia caused by *Clostridium novyi* type B (*oedematiens*) which produces a toxin in necrotic hepatic infarcts. Most cases are seen as sudden onset incidents.

Clinical features: discrete, irregular, pale infarcts on the liver surface (4.98) are characteristic of this acute toxemia. Most frequently seen in areas of endemic

4.98. Infectious necrotic hepatitis ("Black disease") with discrete hepatic infarcts (USA)

4.99. Infectious necrotic hepatitis: subserosal perirenal hemorrhage (USA)

fascioliasis, the larvae of *Fasciola hepatica* are the usual cause of the initial damage. The resulting lesions are then colonized by *Clostridia*, which produce a toxin causing severe depression and rapid death from toxemia. Gross pathology may also include extensive subserosal hemorrhage, shown involving the perirenal area in 4.99. The inner skin surface is dark, hence the disease pseudonym.

Differential diagnosis: other clostridial diseases (pp. 240–242), other causes of sudden death.

Management: rarely are clinical cases seen requiring treatment, but they should respond to antibiotics and NSAIDs. Vaccination is indicated if multiple cases are diagnosed.

Hepatic abscessation

Clinical features: clinical signs include nonspecific pyrexia, anorexia, abdominal pain, and depressed yield. On autopsy hepatic abscesses are usually multiple and vary in size. In this case (4.100) a large, central abscess has ruptured to release creamy pus. Typical causes are an acute rumenitis (4.57), which is followed by hematogenous spread to the neighboring liver, or as sequelae to navel infection or traumatic reticulitis. Such abscesses usually yield *Arcanobacterium pyogenes* on culture, although the initial hepatic colonization is generally by *Fusobacterium necrophorum*. Fattening steers and high-yielding dairy cows are more susceptible owing to their relatively greater intake of concentrate feed. A specific complication of hepatic abscessation is posterior vena cava thrombosis (5.31) or pulmonary thromboembolism (5.32), discussed elsewhere (p. 92).

Differential diagnosis: traumatic reticulitis, abomasal ulceration, peritonitis.

Management: early cases may respond to aggressive antibiotic therapy, but as abscessation tends to become

4.100. Ruptured hepatic abscess at autopsy (USA)

more severe, with an increasing risk of complications, early culling is advised.

Miscellaneous

Lipomatosis (abdominal fat necrosis)

Definition: large lipomatous masses in peritoneal cavity.

Clinical features: a vertical section through the pelvic cavity of an old Angus cow (4.101) shows the rectum surrounded and severely constricted by large areas of fat necrosis, which are firm, dry, and caseous. Such areas, which are also called lipomata, may occur in any part of the omental, mesenteric, and retroperitoneal fat. They may cause chronic progressive bowel obstruction.

4.101. Lipomatosis: vertical section through rectum with constricting lipomata (USA)

However, the majority cause no clinical signs and are an incidental finding during rectal examination when they may be confused with a fetus. Although relatively rare, lipomatosis is considered more common in mature or older Channel Island breeds. Although the etiology is unclear, genetic factors, an excessive intake of soya beans, and persistent pyrexia have been suggested.

Differential diagnosis: abdominal lymphosarcoma, chronic peritonitis with adhesions of abdominal viscera.

Management: lipomatosis cannot be treated.

Rectal prolapse

Clinical features: protrusion of the rectal mucosa is obvious. In 4.102 rectal prolapse had started 24 hours previously, primarily involving the mucosa, which is still fresh and almost undamaged. The second case (4.103) had begun 7 days previously and shows severe lacerations and edema. The only undamaged area is close to the skin–mucosal junction. Rectal prolapse occurs mainly, but not exclusively, in young animals with acute severe, or chronic diarrhea resulting in recurrent tenesmus. Occasionally rectal and vaginal prolapse are seen together, as in this Piedmontese heifer with rectal damage and hemorrhage (4.104). The heifer had a maize-induced tenesmus and rectal prolapse, and vaginal prolapse secondary to dystocia the previous month. Recovery followed induction of a sacral nerve block (alcohol), Buhner suture of the vulvar lips, and dietary correction. Other

4.102. Rectal prolapse of 24 hours' duration. Note perineal blood

4

4.103. Rectal prolapse at 7 days showing multiple lacerations and edema

4.105. Anal edema with mucosal protrusion

predisposing causes of tenesmus are coccidiosis (2.31), babesia (12.43), necrotic enteritis (2.35), and occasionally rabies (9.34).

Management: replace prolapse under epidural analgesia and keep in place with a purse-string suture. Control causes of tenesmus.

Anal edema

Anal edema (4.105) leading to protrusion of the recto-anal mucosa is an occasional iatrogenic result of rectal palpation.

Management: spontaneous recovery is seen within 12–24 hours and no treatment is required.

4.104. Rectal and vaginal prolapse (Italy)

Respiratory disorders

Introduction

Although respiratory diseases have a variety of causes, infectious agents predominate, e.g., infectious bovine rhinotracheitis (IBR) is caused by a herpesvirus that can affect several body systems.

A second group of important respiratory infections is caused by *Pasteurella* spp., usually following exposure of young cattle to stress (hence the alternative name for pasteurellosis, "shipping fever"). Both *Mannheimia haemolytica* serovar 1 and *P. multocida* are normal inhabitants of the upper respiratory tract and in particular the tonsillar crypts. In order to permit colonization of the lungs, stress or a primary viral infection such as bovine virus diarrhea/mucosal disease (BVD/MD), respiratory syncytial virus (RSV), or parainfluenza type 3 (PI-3), must compromise the defense mechanisms of the body.

A third respiratory infection, termed endemic or enzootic calf pneumonia, affects groups of young calves and is of major economic importance. Both viruses (e.g., PI-3, BVD, IBR, RSV, adeno- and rhinoviruses) and mycoplasmas may be primary agents, but the etiology of many outbreaks remains uncertain, since bacterial colonization by *Pasteurella* spp. tends rapidly to supervene. Consequently, the primary virus infection may have been cleared by the time of autopsy. The role of *Chlamydia* is unclear.

Histophilus somni is of major importance as a cause of suppurative pneumonia (9.29), but, having effects on several organ systems, it is presented as infectious thromboembolic meningoencephalitis in Chapter 9.

Respiratory diseases in young cattle are of great economic importance, since their immunity to many etiological agents is poor and vaccination regimes therefore have severe limitations. Antibiotic therapy can be very costly, and recovering cattle often show poor weight gain. Contagious bovine pleuropneumonia (CBPP) is a problem in many developing countries, such as parts of Africa, India, and China, where eradication through a slaughter policy and vaccination programs presents major organizational problems.

Chapter 5 is divided into infectious (viral, bacterial, and other agents) and noninfectious (allergic, iatrogenic, circulatory, and physiological) etiology. Where appropriate, cross-reference is made to other sections for lesions affecting other systems, e.g., both calf diphtheria and laryngeal abscessation (2.42–2.46) are shown in the neonatal chapter, even though they sometimes occur in older animals.

Infectious disorders

Infectious bovine rhinotracheitis (IBR) ("rednose")

Etiology and pathogenesis: IBR is caused by bovine herpesvirus 1 (BHV-1). In addition to respiratory disease, other major syndromes due to BHV-1 include abortion and genital tract infections. BHV-1.1 is the respiratory subtype, BHV-1.2 the genital subtype, and BHV-1.3 the encephalitic subtype. The last-named was recently reclassified as BHV-S, a distinct herpesvirus. *Pasteurella* spp. are common secondary invaders. BHV-1 can cause severe disease in young calves involving pyrexia, ocular and nasal discharge, respiratory distress, and incoordination, leading to convulsions and death.

5.1. Infectious bovine rhinotracheitis (IBR) in neonate (Hereford cross)

5

Clinical features: the common respiratory form of IBR has major clinical signs involving the nostrils (hence the alternative name of "rednose") and the eyes. Feedlot cattle are at particular risk. Within a group of young cattle, several individuals may be affected simultaneously with epiphora and depression. Severely affected animals, such as the crossbred neonate in 5.1, are dull, somnolent, anorexic with a tucked-up belly, and have a mucopurulent nasal discharge, nasal mucosal congestion and lymphadenopathy, and sometimes a harsh cough. The palpebral conjunctivae may be intensely injected or congested in the acute stage (5.2). Characteristic, small, raised, red plaques are visible near the lateral canthus. Secondary infection may lead to a purulent oculonasal discharge (5.3) as well as a typical purulent IBR conjunctivitis, without blepharospasm.

Autopsy examination of this animal (5.4) reveals a severe necrotizing and hemorrhagic laryngotracheitis. Another severe case is shown in 5.5. In severe cases the nasal septum (5.6) sloughs its necrotic mucosa. Epistaxis may follow the rupture of mucosal vessels.

Balanoposthitis can occur with bovine herpesvirus 1 infection (p. 182). In 5.7, the separated vulval lips reveal the multiple, discrete pustules of infectious pustular vulvovaginitis (IPVV). The similarity of the male and female lesions is obvious (compare 10.29).

5.3. IBR with purulent oculonasal discharge

Differential diagnosis: the characteristic signs, pyrexia, and eye lesions especially make diagnosis simple in uncomplicated cases. It is preferable in a field outbreak to attempt virus isolation for confirmation, or demonstration of a rising antibody titer. Bulk milk antibody tests give a simple and inexpensive indication of herd status.

5.2. IBR with severe palpebral congestion

5.4. IBR with severe necrotizing hemorrhagic laryngotracheitis

5.5. IBR with severe purulent tracheitis (USA)

5.8. Pasteurellosis ("shipping fever") severe respiratory distress in calf (Hereford cross)

5.6. IBR nasal septum with necrotic mucosal slough

Management: many cattle only with eye lesions will recover spontaneously, though there is a subsequent risk of poor fertility and an increased abortion rate. Antimicrobial therapy is needed to prevent or treat secondary infections (*Pasteurella*). Breeding cattle, replacement heifers, and calves may be vaccinated from 2 months old with intramuscular or intranasal administration of modified live vaccines. Cattle entering a feedlot should be immunized 2–3 weeks before admission, but the immune response is poorer.

IBR is being successfully eradicated in some European countries by serological testing and either culling reactors or strict maintenance of a two-herd system.

Pasteurellosis ("shipping fever", "transit fever")

Definition: pneumonic pasteurellosis is frequently caused by *Mannheimia haemolytica* serovar 1 biotype A, sometimes by *P. multocida* or *Histophilus somni*, which are all normal inhabitants of the upper respiratory tract. Often pasteurellosis is secondary to respiratory viral infections.

Etiology and pathogenesis: after stress, e.g., transport and/or viral infection, these organisms proliferate rapidly and extend into the trachea, bronchi, and lungs. *A. pyogenes* is a frequent secondary invader.

Clinical features: severe respiratory distress (5.8), with the head and neck extended, open-mouth breathing, and froth on the lips, is obvious in this calf, which died an hour after the photograph was taken. Severe respiratory signs were evident, with dullness and anorexia, pyrexia, and a moist cough. The cranioventral lung fields reveal wheezing sounds on auscultation. An expiratory grunt is possible. Another tucked-up beef steer (5.9) shows severe dyspnea as open-mouth breathing.

At autopsy examination of another calf (5.10), in addition to froth in the major bronchi, the apical and cardiac lobes are typically dark red, slightly swollen, firm, and

5.7. Infectious pustular vulvovaginitis (IPVV) form of bovine herpesvirus infection

5.9. Open-mouth breathing in steer with pasteurellosis

5

5.10.   Pasteurellosis with severe lung changes

contain microabscesses. The diaphragmatic lobes are normal. Such lungs may have fibrin deposits on the pleural surface. Lung changes tend to be symmetrical. In 5.11 the pneumonic areas of the apical and cardiac lobes show scattered, pale yellow abscesses. (See also *H. somni*, 9.29.)

Differential diagnosis: diagnosis depends on bacterial culture from material derived from the lower respiratory tract, or from lung tissue at autopsy. Antibiotic sensitivity testing should be done. Serology is unhelpful in diagnosis.

Management: prompt and aggressive antibiotic therapy should extend well beyond the resolution of clinical signs in affected calves to minimize the development of chronic lung abscessation. NSAIDs are

5.11.   Pasteurellosis with multiple small pulmonary abscesses

important when lung congestion and respiratory signs are severe.

Pasteurella toxoid vaccines are very effective for control, but several doses may be needed in young calves where the immune response is poorer.

Hemorrhagic septicemia

Definition: a severe and frequently fatal septicemic pasteurellosis of cattle caused by *Pasteurella multocida* type B:2 or E:2.

Clinical features: the condition is characterized by sudden severe pyrexia, dyspnea, salivation, hot and painful edematous skin swellings, and submucosal petechiation. It occurs primarily in Asia, Africa, and occasionally parts of Southern Europe and the Middle East. Most outbreaks are in the rainy season in river valleys and deltas.

Diagnosis is readily made on the typical autopsy features of edema, widespread hemorrhages, and often hemopericardium. Pneumonic changes, except for hemorrhages, are minor.

Differential diagnosis: pneumonic pasteurellosis (5.8–5.11), Rinderpest [eradicated worldwide 2010] (12.9–12.15), anthrax (12.63), acute salmonellosis.

Management: prompt chemotherapy (sulfonamides, tetracyclines) is effective. Prevention is by vaccination twice yearly, preferably with the oil-adjuvant or alum-precipitated bacterin.

Endemic (enzootic) calf pneumonia

Definition: endemic calf pneumonia is a broad and ill-defined entity, covering infectious pulmonary disease in young cattle that is unassociated with transport stress, but frequently related to overcrowded conditions indoors or in yards.

Etiology and pathogenesis: the etiology and epidemiology involve a wide range of viral and bacterial pathogens (see "Introduction").

Clinical features: the first signs are often serous ocular discharge and mild conjunctivitis. Later, a secondary infection (often *Pasteurella* spp.) can cause a bilateral mucopurulent nasal discharge (5.12). Some calves (5.13) develop a "sweaty" coat with damp and matted hair. Similar coat changes can also be seen in some healthy, fast-growing calves on a high-concentrate feed. However, coughing, with or without dyspnea, is often pronounced. Many animals in a group will be pyrexic and anorexic. Deaths may be seen within a few days of the onset of obvious clinical signs.

At autopsy the lungs contain pink-gray or purplish areas of consolidation typically in the apical and cardiac lobes and usually (5.14) without overlying fibrin. A cross-section of this lung (5.15) shows an edematous

5.12. Endemic calf pneumonia showing mucopurulent nasal discharge

5.15. Endemic calf pneumonia: cross-section of lung

consolidated pneumonic area ventrally and normal pink lung isolated at the top. *Mycoplasma dispar.* was isolated. Secondary infection can lead to pulmonary abscessation. Respiratory syncytial virus (RSV) lungs typically show areas of emphysematous bullae (A) and patchy consolidation (B), which, as in this calf (5.16), are often in the caudal (diaphragmatic) lobes, although all lung lobes may potentially be affected. Note the typical grossly distended emphysematous changes causing rounding of the lung margin with RSV.

Differential diagnosis: several viruses as well as a secondary bacterial invader may be involved. Serology and autopsy features aid differentiation.

5.13. "Sweaty coat" in endemic calf pneumonia

Management: proper housing and ventilation, adequate colostral intake as neonate, individual pens until 2–3 months old for milk-fed calves; avoid mixing multiple age groups in same air-space, as well as mixed-source calves with varying immune and disease status. Provide dry, draught-free, but well-ventilated housing. Replace straw bedding frequently (e.g., every 4–6 weeks). Calfhood vaccination, following identification of the causative agent is effective control. Whole group antibiotic therapy is effective in outbreaks.

5.14. Endemic calf pneumonia with lung consolidation

5.16. RSV calf pneumonia with (A) emphysematous bullae, and (B) patchy consolidation

5

5.17.   Chronic suppurative pneumonia in beef heifer

Chronic suppurative pneumonia

Chronic pneumonia is often suppurative, and many organisms can be involved. Cattle of all ages can be affected. The dull beef heifer in 5.17 shows typical signs of chronic pneumonia, including loss of condition, an extended tongue, head and neck, and severe dyspnea, leading to froth on the lips. A profuse mucopurulent nasal discharge is also often seen in chronic suppurative pneumonia, as in a 7-year-old Holstein cow (5.18), together with a persistent cough. Autopsy examination (5.19) shows darkened areas of consolidation (A), emphysematous bullae (B), and abscessation (C). (See also 9.29.)

Management: prolonged aggressive antibiotic therapy (e.g., 1–2 weeks) is sometimes effective in early stages but, after this, most cases must be culled as incurable.

Contagious bovine pleuropneumonia ("lung sickness")

Definition and etiology: caused by *Mycoplasma mycoides mycoides*, contagious bovine pleuropneumonia

5.19.   Chronic suppurative pneumonia with (A) consolidation, (B) emphysematous bullae, and (C) abscessation (USA)

(CBPP) is a highly contagious pulmonary disease that is often accompanied by pleurisy. It continues to be rampant in many parts of Africa (at least 30 countries), India, and China, and minor outbreaks occur in the Middle East. CBPP was seen in Italy 1990–93 and in 1997 it occurred in Portugal.

Clinical features: CBPP infection arises predominantly from droplet inhalation in susceptible cattle, and occasionally from ingestion of infected urine or placentae. In susceptible herds the morbidity may reach 100%, the mortality 50%, and 50% of the survivors may become carriers. The main autopsy features are a severe serofibrinous pleurisy (5.20) and fibrinonecrotic pneumonia. In 5.21 note the interlobular septa (A) massively distended by fibrinous exudates, creating a marbling effect. The darker areas of lung (B) are undergoing consolidation and necrosis. Chronic lung lesions include large sequestra containing viable organisms, which act as an important reservoir of infection. In 5.22 a large subpleural sequestrum (A) is seen to the left of a large pleuritic lesion (B). The material can be projected as an infectious aerosol by carrier cattle which may be clinically normal,

5.18.   Chronic suppurative pneumonia in cow (Holstein, 7 years old)

5.20.   Contagious bovine pleuropneumonia (CBPP) with pleurisy and fibrinonecrotic pneumonia

5.21. CBPP with marbling appearance of lungs

i.e. overt clinical signs may not be apparent despite damaged lungs.

Differential diagnosis: diagnosis is readily made on clinical signs, CF test, and autopsy features. Acute pasteurellosis (5.9–5.11) is the major differential.

Management: CBPP has been eradicated, using a compulsory slaughter policy, from North America, most of Europe (except the Iberian peninsula and parts of the Balkans), and Australia. Eradication is difficult because some infected animals become carriers and the efficacy of available vaccines is relatively poor. In most countries all outbreaks of CBPP must be notified to the central animal health authorities. Treatment is limited to endemic areas of CBPP. Elsewhere quarantine, blood testing, and immunization with an attenuated vaccine can restrict disease spread.

Tuberculosis

Etiology and pathogenesis: bovine tuberculosis is caused by *Mycobacterium bovis* and is transmissible to

5.23. Tuberculosis lymph node with caseous granules

humans, usually via infected milk. Bovine organs commonly infected with tuberculosis include the lungs, alimentary tract and udder.

Clinical features: most cases of TB are identified and culled before clinical signs are seen. In advanced cases respiratory TB leads to a chronic moist cough, later dyspnea, and abnormal sounds on auscultation. Lymphadenopathy, progressive emaciation, and lethargy follow. Lung lesions have areas of yellow-orange pus that frequently become caseous (5.23). The lung shows numerous nodules, one opened to demonstrate the cheese-like contents, and a regional lymph node is held by a gloved hand. Brownish "grape-like" masses may adhere to the pleura (5.24). Gross granulomatous nodules may develop beneath the intestinal mucosa (5.25).

Diagnostic tests: TB skin test and ELISA serology.

Management: while many countries have now largely eradicated the disease, tuberculosis acquired from cattle remains a major human health hazard in parts of Africa,

5.22. CBPP: (A) subpleural sequestrum, and (B) pleurisy

5.24. TB "grapes" on pleura

5.25. Tuberculosis: submucosal intestinal granulomatous nodules (USA)

5.27. Maturing lungworm larvae in bronchi

the Indian subcontinent, and the Far East, where the slow, chronic nature of the infection makes early clinical diagnosis difficult. Where a test and slaughter policy is not feasible, test (every 3 months) and segregation of reactors is an alternative. In some countries a wildlife reservoir (e.g., badger in UK and possum in New Zealand) has markedly slowed down eradication of the disease.

Lungworm infection (verminous bronchitis, "husk", "hoose")

Definition: a lower respiratory tract infection caused by *Dictyocaulus viviparus*.

Pathogenesis and clinical features: the cattle lungworm causes bronchitis and pneumonia in young animals exposed to infective larvae during the first grazing season. The problem is primarily seen in the temperate areas of northwestern Europe. Clinical disease does not usually occur until the late summer and autumn. Early (prepatent) infection is seen as tachypnea, partial anorexia, and marked weight loss. In later stages a persistent cough develops ("husk"), and the calf tends to stand with its head and neck extended (5.26), owing to bronchial irritation from the presence

of the patent forms of *D. viviparus*. A characteristic late feature is the development of a chronic, nonsuppurative, eosinophilic granulomatous pneumonia, primarily in the caudal lobes of the lung. Considerable weight loss results, and clinically recovering cases still show reduced weight gain. Autopsy examination of a severe case (5.27) shows large numbers of maturing larvae in the bronchi and bronchioles. Reinfection can occur in adult cattle (usually in dairy cows in the autumn) in the form of an extensive eosinophilic bronchitis. Primary infection also occurs in adult dairy cattle resulting in pronounced weight loss.

Diagnosis: larvae may be demonstrated in the feces or oronasal mucus of advanced cases, while serology can confirm exposure, but the epidemiology and clinical signs, taken together, are often characteristic.

Management: affected cattle should be given a suitable anthelmintic, and either housed or moved onto a clean pasture. Their old pasture remains infected until summer of the following year. Improve diet to restore lost weight. Strategic anthelmintic therapy (either boluses or repeated dosing) controls lungworm well at that time, but has no long-term protective effect. Optimal prophylaxis is use of an oral irradiated larval vaccine (two doses in the first season, 6 and 4 weeks before turn-out). Boosted immunity derived from subsequent natural exposure can be diminished by concurrent anthelmintic therapy, which should therefore be carefully planned.

Noninfectious disorders

Atypical interstitial pneumonia (bovine pulmonary emphysema, enzootic bovine adenomatosis, "fog fever", "panters")

Definition: an acute hypersensitivity or allergic respiratory disease syndrome, more commonly seen in adult cattle, typically causing pulmonary edema, congestion, interstitial emphysema, and alveolar changes.

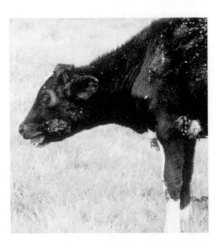

5.26. Lungworm infection ("husk"): coughing calf

5.28. Atypical interstitial pneumonia ("fog fever") in cow (Hereford)

Pathogenesis: it occurs predominantly in groups of heavy adult beef cattle, and, to a lesser extent, in dairy cattle and typically follows 5–10 days after a change from bare grazing onto lush pastures in the autumn, although occasional outbreaks are seen in the spring. Increased levels of nitrogenous fertilizer may be involved in some cases. The amino acid, D,L-tryptophan, the levels of which are high in lush autumn pastures, is thought to be a significant cause of this type of pneumonia, the actual toxic agent being 3-methylindole, a metabolite of D,L-tryptophan that is produced in the rumen.

Clinical features: severe respiratory distress (5.28) is seen, with frothing of saliva, and open-mouth breathing. Moderate exercise, such as moving off the lush pasture, can precipitate severe dyspnea and sometimes collapse and death, as occurred in this case. In some cases subcutaneous emphysema is seen along the back from the withers. The lungs of acute cases (5.29) are heavy, fail to collapse, and have extensive areas of edema and emphysema (A), some of which may form large bullae.

Differential diagnosis: pasteurellosis (5.9–5.11), O–P toxicity (13.26).

Management: cattle should be removed from suspect pastures as soon as possible but with extreme caution to avoid further respiratory distress. Some new cases may nevertheless occur. NSAIDs are important for treatment, and both diuretics and prophylactic antibiotics may be given. Control is by dietary management through slow introduction to lush pastures. Prophylactic feeding of monensin or lasalocid may also be effective.

Aspiration pneumonia (inhalation pneumonia)

Etiology and pathogenesis: inhalation of foreign material such as fluid drenches, or of rumen contents following bloat or occasionally during general anesthesia commonly causes a severe and often fatal pneumonia with pulmonary necrosis. Predisposing causes include abnormal head posture, struggling, bellowing, cleft palate (neonatal calves), and pharyngeal abscessation or neoplasia.

The typical pneumonia is predominantly in the anteroventral parts of the lungs. The right thoracic wall has been removed from a Holstein cow (5.30) to show the effects of accidental aspiration of mineral oil (liquid paraffin) about 60 hours previously. The entire surface of the visible pleura covering the lungs appears greasy as a result of oil leakage through ruptured bullae. Severe interlobular edema and emphysema are evident. Affected lobes may also reveal congestion and early necrosis. Foreign body aspiration (drenches, rumen fluid) is frequently fatal within 48–72 hours.

Management: if aspiration has occurred, the animal should be kept quiet and given NSAIDs and broad-spectrum antibiotic prophylaxis. The prognosis is poor in all cases.

5.29. Atypical interstitial pneumonia: lungs in acute case with edema and emphysema (A) (USA)

5.30. Aspiration pneumonia: right lung *in situ* with mineral oil, edema, and emphysema (USA)

5

5.31. Localized caudal vena caval thrombosis in pulmonary thromboembolism (Canada)

5.33. Renal infarction (A, recent; B, older infarcts) with septic emboli in PTE-CVC (Canada)

Pulmonary thromboembolism (caudal vena caval thrombosis) (PTE-CVC)

Pathogenesis: PTE-CVC affects animals of all ages. The complex etiology of the dramatic syndrome of pulmonary thromboembolism, PTE-CVC can be a consequence of hepatic abscessation, often from navel infections or rumenitis, or can result from an earlier pulmonary disease. In some cases a localized caudal vena caval thrombosis develops (5.31). The hemostat holds the wall of the caudal vena cava. Septic emboli may seed the lungs following bacteremia and septicemia (5.32), and may result from a primary respiratory infection. Septic emboli may spread to other organs, and renal infarction (5.33) is common. The dark areas (A) in the renal cortex are recent infarcts; the paler areas (B) are older. Pulmonary arterial lesions can cause thromboembolism, aneurysm formation, and severe intrabronchial hemorrhage, hemoptysis, anemia, and melena from swallowed blood. In an ultimately fatal hemoptysis resulting from PTE-CVC (5.34), frothy arterial blood is seen on the muzzle of this cow and in pools among the straw bedding.

5.34. Fatal hemoptysis in pulmonary thromboembolism

Management: dietary control measures to prevent the development of rumenitis and acidosis. Control of respiratory disease and other bacterial infections. The acute clinical case cannot be effectively treated, but low-grade epistaxis and pyrexia may respond to antibiotic therapy.

5.32. Pulmonary thromboembolism (PTE-CVC) with septic emboli

5.35. Brisket disease in heifer with severe edema (Hereford) (Colorado, USA)

Brisket disease (altitude sickness, high mountain disease)

Pathogenesis and clinical features: brisket disease results from congestive cardiac failure at high altitudes (usually above 2 200 meters), where impairment of the circulatory or respiratory system overcomes the cardiac reserve capacity and causes chronic physiological hypoxia. Though individual susceptibility is great, both sexes and all ages (but predominantly <1 year) and most breeds can be affected. For unknown reasons, grazing of locoweed increases the prevalence. The Hereford heifer (5.35) from Colorado, USA, shows pronounced submandibular and presternal edema, depression, and dehydration.

Differential diagnosis: other causes of congestive cardiac failure.

Management: movement with due caution to a lower altitude, avoidance of locoweed.

5

Cardiovascular disorders

Introduction

This chapter is short not because cardiovascular disorders are uncommon, but because many conditions are illustrated in other chapters. Three basic cardiac syndromes encompass most disorders: the first is congestive cardiac failure, which may result from valvular disease (6.4), myocardial or pericardial disease (6.5–6.8), hypertension, or congenital defects which produce shunts (1.30–1.32). Secondly, and less commonly, acute heart failure can result from tachyarrhythmia caused by a nutritional deficiency myopathy (e.g., copper or selenium), electrocution or lightning strike (classified under nervous disorders, 9.41–9.44), or bradycardia due to plant poisoning by *Solanum*, *Trisetum* and *Lantana* species, all of which can induce myocardial changes (13.13–13.16). Thirdly, peripheral circulatory failure can result from vasodilatation and a reduced circulating blood volume as in septic shock (e.g., acute gangrenous mastitis and acute metritis), or endotoxic shock from a peracute coliform mastitis (11.4–11.9). Peripheral circulatory failure can also be due to hematogenic failure as a result of severe hemorrhage (see 5.34), or as a consequence of neonatal calf diarrhea (2.16–2.24).

Congestive cardiac failure

Definition and pathogenesis: in congestive cardiac failure reduced myocardial contractility results in reduced cardiac output and pulmonary edema when the left ventricle fails, or ascites and/or pitting edema in right-sided congestive failure, when circulatory impairment impedes venous return.

Clinical features: following right-sided failure of the heart to pump an adequate volume of blood to the lungs, jugular venous distension ("jugular cording") may be marked as seen in the Friesian cow in 6.1. The cow was dull, pyrexic, and developed a chronic cough as a result of passive venous congestion. Poor venous return in the Limousin cross bull (6.2) resulted in the development of a dependent edema in the submandibular, presternal, and ventral abdominal and preputial areas.

6.1. Congestive cardiac failure: jugular venous distension in cow (Friesian)

Differential diagnosis: ventral edema due to circulatory failure should be distinguished from a transient peripartum udder edema which is normal in dairy cows (see 11.55), and from subcutaneous edema (3.1, 3.2).

Management: largely symptomatic, including diuretics (furosemide or chlorothiazide); attempted identification of primary cause. Most cases must be culled.

6.2. Congestive cardiac failure in bull, with extensive edema (Limousin cross)

6.3.   Vegetative endocarditis: proliferative masses surrounding right AV valve

6.5.   Septic pericarditis in bull with (A) fibrosed epicardium, and (B) sternum (Charolais)

Vegetative or nodular endocarditis

Pathogenesis and clinical features: another cause of congestive cardiac failure, bovine endocarditis may involve septicemia and chronic bacteremia resulting from a remote focus, such as an infected joint or the umbilicus. Characteristic signs include weight loss, drop in yield, exercise intolerance, dependent edema, tachycardia, and heart murmur. Alternatively, the lesion may develop slowly in adult cattle, which remain asymptomatic, and manifest no evidence of bacterial infection (endocardiosis). In bacterial endocarditis, the tricuspid (right AV) and mitral (left AV) valves are most commonly affected.

Submandibular and ventral edema are evident in a poor Friesian cow with a history of claw sepsis, which rapidly went into right heart failure. A transverse section of the heart shows massive lesions of vegetative endocarditis (6.3) in the right atrioventricular valve.

The Guernsey cow in 6.4 (see also 3.68) developed a large abscess involving the left subcutaneous abdominal vein (milk vein), which caused severe valvular endocarditis and death. Contrast the pendulant midline mass (3.69) which is a massive fibroma well separated from the milk veins. Some cases that occur in young calves may have prominent valvular nodules from which *Mannheimia haemolytica* serovar 1 and α-hemolytic streptococci can be

isolated, suggesting that the original infection involved the respiratory tract. Environmental streptococci, including *S. uberis*, have been isolated from clusters of cases where heifers were introduced into dairy herds under high-stress conditions.

Management: antibiotic therapy seems to stop development of lesions in early stages, and animals may well adapt to the valvular leakage. Preventive steps include control of calfhood respiratory disease, improved integration of first lactation heifers into dairy herds, and reduction of the risk of septic foci.

Septic pericarditis and myocarditis

Pathogenesis: commonly follows traumatic reticuloperitonitis, less commonly from hematogenous spread.

Clinical features: septic pericarditis is usually a sequel to penetration of the pericardial sac by a wire that has migrated from the reticulum through the diaphragm (see "Traumatic reticulitis", p. 69). Congestive cardiac failure is the result of reduced contractility. In the Charolais bull in 6.5 a massive volume of yellow pus ("scrambled egg" appearance) fills the pericardial sac. The surface (A) below the pus is the thickened, partly fibrosed epicardium. The

6.4.   Massive abscess in left subcutaneous abdominal vein

6.6.   Septic pericarditis

6.7. Myocarditis with foreign body (wire) embedded

6.8. Fatal myocardial abscessation following hematogenous route

thickness of the pericardial wall can be judged from the depth of the sternum (B). Another illustration of septic pericarditis is seen in 6.6, with organized purulent exudate adhering to the epicardial surface as well as pericardium.

Heart failure may result from migration of the foreign body (wire, A) into the myocardium itself (6.7). Ventral edema is often a sequel to septic pericarditis caused by traumatic reticulitis.

The absence of a septic track from the reticulum through the diaphragm to the pericardium and heart in another case (6.8) indicates that fatal myocardial abscessation can sometimes arise through hematogenous infection. In this cow (6.8), in which the original septic focus was a septic pedal arthritis, the abscess (opened) involves the papillary muscles and myocardium.

Cardiac tamponade due to massive sudden accumulation of blood in the pericardial sac (4.68) following tire wire penetration from the reticulum results either in sudden death (as here) or congestive cardiac failure.

Management: treatment of individual cases is rarely successful.

Control: see "Traumatic reticulitis" (p. 69)

6

Chapter 7

Locomotor disorders

Lower limb and digit

Introduction

In dairy cattle, approximately 80% of all lameness originates in the foot, most often in one of the hind feet, arising
in the lateral hind claw in the majority of cases. In addition to significant welfare implications, lameness is a
major cause of economic loss, as affected animals lose
weight rapidly, yields fall and, in protracted cases, fertility
is affected. There is also increased culling, and considerable sums of money are spent on treatment and preventive
hoof trimming. The severe pain associated with lameness
(7.1) is seen as an arched back, front legs forward and
apart to take increased weight, and head lowered to bring
the center of gravity forward and away from the painful
left hind limb. Although accurate figures are not available,
lameness in beef cattle has a lower incidence and less
economic importance. Many etiological factors are
involved, including excessive standing, especially on hard,
unyielding tracks and surfaces; rough handling when
moving cattle; feet kept continually wet in corrosive slurry;
reduced horn growth at calving; and high-concentrate/
low-fiber feeds leading to acidosis. All of these factors
can precipitate laminitis/coriosis, the consequences of
which are abnormal horn growth and hoof wear, softening

7.1. Lame cow

of the sole horn, dropping of the distal phalanx within
the hoof, and a weakening and widening of the white line,
all of which predispose to digital lameness.

This chapter illustrates the common foot lesions in cattle,
namely white line abscess, sole ulcer, interdigital necrobacillosis, interdigital skin hyperplasia, and digital dermatitis.
Complications of these primary conditions may produce
deeper digital infections, often involving the navicular
bursa and, eventually, the pedal (distal interphalangeal)

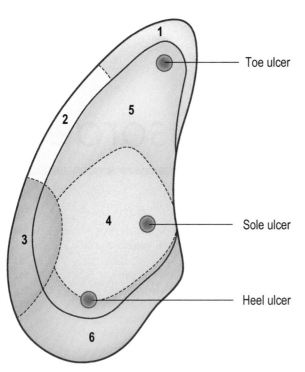

7.2.   Zones of the foot

Toe ulcer

Sole ulcer

Heel ulcer

7.3.   White line disease in right lateral claw

joint. Flexor tendon rupture or coronary band abscessation may result. The final section deals with laminitis/coriosis. Digital lesions due to systemic disease, e.g., foot-and-mouth (12.7) are described in the relevant chapters. The zones of the foot, as defined by the International Ruminant Lameness Symposium, are shown in 7.2, and this nomenclature will be used in the following sections.

Disorders of the sole and axial wall

White line disorders

Definition: the white line is the cemented junction between the sole horn and the hoof wall (zones 1 and 2 in 7.2). It consists of nontubular horn, and as a consequence it is much weaker than the tubular horn of the wall and sole. Disorders of the corium lead to the production of defective white line cement, which predisposes to separation of the sole from the wall and allows entry of small stones, debris, dirt, and infection. Stones in particular act as a wedge, further separating wall from sole. Infection reaching the corium produces pus, the pressure of which causes pain and subsequent lameness. Some cases are thought to arise from an internal sterile inflammation of the corium.

Clinical features: early cases of white line disease are seen as a yellow discoloration (caused by serum) or reddening (caused by hemorrhage) of the white line cement. 7.3 illustrates white line hemorrhage in zone 2 in the right (lateral) claw, hemorrhage at the sole ulcer site

(zone 4 left claw), and areas of yellow discoloration in both claws. In more advanced cases (7.4) a fissure develops in the defective white line allowing the penetration of stones and other debris, which then act as a wedge, producing further white line separation. Infection reaching the corium may track either across the sole, or proximally along the laminae, as in 7.5, to discharge at the coronary band. The abaxial white line of the hind lateral

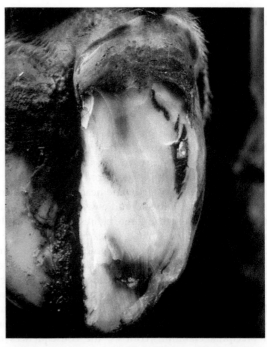

7.4.   Fissure in claw in white line disease with foreign body

7.5. Purulent discharge at coronary band following ascending white line disease

7.7. Removal of under-run sole horn with new horn (A) and hemorrhage at B (compare 7.6)

claw is most frequently involved, especially zone 3 toward the heel, as it represents a mechanical stress line between the rigid hoof wall and the movement of the flexible heel during locomotion.

A variety of white line abscesses are seen, depending on both the initial site of penetration of the infection and on the direction of spread. On the left claw of 7.6 light-grayish pus is exuding from the point of entry of infection at the white line near the toe. Pus has tracked under the sole horn, leading to separation of the horn from the underlying corium. Lameness was pronounced. In 7.7 the under-run sole has been removed to expose new sole horn, developing as a layer of creamy-white tissue (A) in the center of the sole and against the edge of the trimmed

horn. The hemorrhagic area (B) at the white line is the original point of entry of infection. Progressively deeper penetration of infection occurs in untreated cases. In 7.8, another sole view, the corium has been eroded to expose the tip of the pedal bone (A). This resulted in severe lameness, although the cow eventually made a full recovery. In 7.9 a white line lesion had tracked from the sole dorsally along the laminar corium, then the papillary corium to discharge at the coronary band. Removal of the under-run hoof wall revealed a brown necrotic line. This has permitted drainage. A wooden block has been glued onto the sound claw to rest the affected digit. Although this cow walked soundly within 3 weeks, more than 12 months elapsed before sufficient horn had grown down from the coronet fully to repair the damaged hoof.

Differential diagnosis: punctured (FB) sole, bruised sole, sole ulcer, fracture of distal phalanx, vertical wall fissure.

7.6. Pus exuding from white line near toe

7.8. Exposure of pedal bone following erosion of sole horn

7.9. Removal of hoof wall to allow drainage of ascending white line infection

7.10. Axial wall fissure

Management: white line disorders are primarily a defect of the corium leading to the production of defective cement. Coriosis may be the result of a range of factors including trauma (e.g., prolonged standing due to poor cubicle comfort, or prolonged feeding and milking times), diet (rumen acidosis leads to reduced biotin synthesis and the production of defective white line cement), and environment. An increased incidence of white line separation and abscess formation may occur when cattle are forced to walk rapidly along rough surfaces or tracks where there are small, sharp flints. It may also be a consequence of softening of the hoof, e.g., excessively wet conditions underfoot. Both reduced horn growth and increased pedal bone movement at calving predispose to bruising of the corium, with an increased incidence of white line defects and sole ulcers seen 2–3 months later when the defective horn has reached the bearing surface of the sole.

Axial wall fissure and penetration

Definition: the fissure is a defect of the white line where it passes dorsally along the axial wall towards the interdigital cleft. The axial groove horn is very thin (1–2 mm) and therefore predisposed to foreign body penetration.

Clinical features: most cases of fissure here (7.10) are seen as an impaction of the white line with black debris, often with under-running of adjacent horn. Pain and lameness are a result of the detached axial wall moving on the underlying corium. A foreign body penetrating this region resulted in a localized septic laminitis (7.28) at A, with secondary interdigital swelling and necrosis.

Differential diagnosis: interdigital FB, interdigital dermatitis.

Management: removing under-run horn treats individual cases. Predisposing factors are as in white line disorders, although wet environmental conditions are thought to be particularly important, and digital dermatitis in the interdigital space, leading to defective horn production from the coronary band, may be a further cause.

Sole overgrowth

Definition: the central sole area, namely zone 4 beneath the flexor tuberosity of the pedal bone, should be non-weightbearing. However, it is not uncommon for a wedge of sole to grow out from zone 3 to 4 to become the major weightbearing area of the sole. This is especially the case if the wall becomes worn away, e.g., from excessive standing on concrete, and the sole becomes weightbearing. Trauma to the solar corium beneath the flexor tuberosity of the pedal bone stimulates increased horn growth, but the sole horn produced is often softer and hemorrhage may be seen. Sole ulcers may then develop beneath this wedge.

Clinical features: the lateral (left) claw in 7.11 is much larger than the medial claw, and a wedge of overgrown sole horn (A) which has become the major weightbearing surface is growing across towards the medial claw. This wedge predisposes the animal to sole bruising and/or sole ulcers (see 7.13, 7.34). A plantar view is shown in 7.12. The black areas on the heels are early heel erosions (7.67). In front feet sole overgrowth is more commonly seen in the medial claw.

Management: thought to be a consequence of coriosis/laminitis resulting from excess standing, sole overgrowth is seen especially in heifers 6–12 weeks after calving. Heifers that have been reared in straw yards prior to calving have a thinner sole which is more prone to bruising when they move onto concrete postpartum. The problem is exacerbated by other causes of coriosis such as poor cubicle/free stall comfort and an inappropriate diet. Corrective trimming, possibly repeated, to return normal weight distribution to the wall is required.

7.11. Sole overgrowth with lateral claw, showing grossly overgrown abaxial wall and sole wedge (A)

7.13. Sole ulcer in (left) exungulated claw (A) and (right) hemorrhage at heel ulcer site (B)

Sole ulcers ("Rusterholz")

Definition: an ulcer is a defect in the horn at zone 4 exposing the underlying corium, and like white line disorders, sole ulceration originates from a defective corium. Heel and toe ulcers are discussed in the next section. Sole ulcers are the most common and are typically found on the axial aspect of the sole in zone 4, beneath the flexor tuberosity of the pedal bone. 7.13 shows two exungulated claws, the left with severe hemorrhage in the corium at the sole (A) which could develop into a sole ulcer, and the right with hemorrhage at the heel ulcer site (B).

Clinical features: in the digit in 7.12 (a plantar view) the wall has been worn down to the level of the sole or lower, and a wedge of sole horn (A) is growing from the axial aspect of the right (lateral) claw towards the left claw. This wedge becomes a major weightbearing surface and transmits excess weight to the sole corium, causing hemorrhage, bruising, and eventually defective horn formation. Note also the heel erosion (B). Another cow (7.14)

7.12. Sole ulcer with wedge of sole horn

7.14. Sole ulcer: discrete area of hemorrhage

7.15. Claw in 7.14 further pared to reveal sole ulcer

shows that when such a sole wedge is pared away, a discrete area of sole hemorrhage is revealed in the right (lateral) claw. Note the reddening of the white line in the same claw, indicative of coriosis/laminitis, and also that both claws are overgrown. Further paring and removal of the hemorrhagic horn (7.15) revealed under-run horn and necrosis characteristic of a sole ulcer. Some sole ulcers (7.16) develop a large, protruding mass of granulation tissue. The longitudinal section of another case (7.17) illustrates a mild, chronic ulcer in its characteristic site beneath the flexor tuberosity at the sole–heel junction. The sole horn has been perforated (A) and inflammatory changes have tracked up towards the insertion of the deep flexor tendon. The heel horn is slightly under-run (B) and there is laminitic hemorrhage (coriosis) at the toe (C). In some longer standing cases a bony enlargement of the plantar surface of the flexor tuberosity exacerbates disruption of the corium. Sole ulcers are typically found on the lateral claws of hind feet and, less frequently, on the

7.16. Protruding granulation tissue in sole ulcer

7.17. Sole ulcer (longitudinal section) at typical site

medial claws of front feet. Often the lateral digits of both hind feet are involved to a different extent. More extensive damage to the corium means ulcers heal more slowly than a white line abscess or an under-run sole (7.7).

Differential diagnosis: solar foreign body penetration and abscessation.

Management: coriosis is the primary defect, and hence many of the factors leading to white line disease can also produce sole ulcers. It is now thought that excessive standing especially leads to a high incidence of sole ulcers and sudden sharp turns are important for white line disease. Treatment of individual cases involves paring away all under-run horn around the ulcer, removing excess granulation tissue, and minimizing weightbearing to allow new horn to be produced in the defective site. This can be achieved by paring the affected claw to transfer weight onto the sound claw, and/or by the application of a shoe to the sound claw.

Heel ulcers

Definition: heel ulcers occur in the center of the rear sole, at the junction of zones 4 and 6, where the heel horn joins the sole horn, and are shown as areas of hemorrhage in the exungulated right claw in 7.13. Toe ulcers occur at zone 5.

Clinical features: heel ulcers are seen as a small black track (A), seen on the left claw of 7.18 penetrating the sole horn caudally. An area of adjacent dark under-run horn can be seen at B. Removal of overlying horn may lead to the disappearance of small lesions, but in other cases the track leads into a typically deep abscess cavity in the central heel area. In some cases the lesion discharges at the heel, but the depth of the abscess means that this sequel is by no means as common as in sole ulcers or white line disorders. Heel ulcers commonly occur with sole ulcers, although they are more frequently found on the medial claw of hind feet and the lateral claw of fore feet than sole ulcers. In 7.19 a deep heel ulcer

7.18. Heel ulcer (A) shown by small black track

(A) is in the center of the right claw and a more superficial sole ulcer (B) is on the axial aspect of the left claw, where there is also extensive white line separation and heel horn erosion. Their etiology is not understood but pinching of the corium between cartilaginous changes in the pedal suspensory apparatus above and the hoof of the sole beneath may be the cause.

Differential diagnosis: as for sole ulcer.

Management: for both conditions remove all damaged horn and minimize weightbearing on the affected claw. Control by identifying initial causes of coriosis.

Toe ulcers

Definition: toe ulcers, combined with white line lesions at zone 5 on the axial wall, may arise from excess hoof wear and are common sequelae of over trimming or incorrect hoof paring.

Clinical features: they may present as larger areas of hemorrhage in zone 5 (7.20) or more commonly simply as a softening of the sole, as in 7.21. Note how the hoof wall has been worn away at the toe, and the presence of early subsolar hemorrhage in 7.21. Frequently seen when

7.19. Heel ulcer (A) on medial (right) claw plus sole ulcer (B), white line hemorrhage and heel horn erosion (slurry heel) on left claw

7.20. Toe ulcer with extensive hemorrhage

heifers and young bulls are introduced into a dairy herd without prior acclimatization to concrete, they appear to be related to trauma and excessive wear. Both front and hind feet may be affected. Excess sole wear is becoming a major problem in some herds, and has led to a suggestion that the frequency, or the extent, of hoof trimming should be reduced.

Differential diagnosis: white line disease, toe necrosis.

Management: improved housing and acclimatization to environment.

Toe necrosis (osteomyelitis of distal phalanx)

Definition: abscess at the toe leading to secondary infection of the apex of the pedal (distal phalangeal) bone. Often a sequel to a toe ulcer (7.21). In the UK a high incidence is seen in herds where digital dermatitis is poorly controlled and most cases in dairy cows are

7.21. Excess wear has lead to total erosion of the wall at the toe and exposure of corium (not visible)

7

7.22. Toe necrosis showing typical dorsal rotation of affected digit

infected with treponemes indistinguishable from those causing digital dermatitis.

Clinical features: the condition occurs in both dairy cows and in feedlot cattle, and may be associated with excess wear leading to thinning of the horn at the toe. Dairy cows walk with the affected foot forward to relieve pain in the toe, and this typically leads to overgrowth of horn, seen on the medial toe of the right hind foot of 7.22. Note the predisposing poor hygiene underfoot. In another cleaned foot in 7.23 much of the under-run sole and wall at the toe has largely been removed to reveal a black necrotic area tracking up under the dorsal wall. The lesion invariably has a pronounced putrid smell, rarely present in other hoof disorders. The necrotic tip of the pedal bone may be palpated. In a cross-section of another digit (7.24) the apex of the pedal bone has clearly been eroded at A, dry fecal debris is impacted into the residual cavity at the toe, and gray areas of necrotic pedal bone are visible. Marked osteoporosis and reduced pedal bone density may be evident with toe necrosis, a feature that is not seen in other non-healing hoof lesions associated with digital dermatitis.

Management: thorough removal of all under-run horn, debridement, cleaning, and packing with antibiotic will result in recovery of a few cases, but many need more

7.24. Toe necrosis in cross-section with erosion of pedal bone

radical treatment such as amputation of either the osteomyelitic and necrotic tip of the pedal bone, or of the whole claw. Many conventionally treated lesions fail to heal and recur a few months later, although some are not severely lame, and regular trimming of the affected toe may allow continued production.

Foreign body penetration of the sole

Definition: penetration of the sole by a foreign body allowing access of infection to the corium and subsequent under-run sole and abscess formation.

Clinical features: the most common foreign bodies are nails, stones, and cast teeth. In 7.25 a metal staple is firmly impacted in the sole, toward the heel. Unless the foreign body penetrates the sole horn, leading to infection and under-run corium, lameness is relatively mild. In 7.26 a portion of nail has penetrated the sole horn on the axial aspect of the white line, carrying infection into the corium. In 7.27 the superficial under-run horn and adjoining wall have been removed to provide drainage

7.23. Toe necrosis

7.25. Foreign body (metallic staple) in sole

7.26.   Foreign body perforating sole near axial white line

and to expose the new sole (A) developing beneath. In the center (B) is the sensitive corium. Foreign body penetration can also occur near the axial groove (7.28) as the wall horn is thinnest here, leading to secondary interdigital swelling and necrosis, and a septic laminitis. Sole puncture at the toe can cause osteomyelitis of the distal phalanx or pedal bone (7.23, 7.24).

Management: removal of foreign body and paring of surrounding under-run horn to permit optimal drainage. If the foreign body has penetrated into deeper tissues of the heel, long-term and aggressive parenteral antibiotics are indicated.

7.27.   Sole of 7.25 pared to permit drainage

7.28.   Foreign body penetration near axial groove

False sole

Definition: a "false sole" occurs when a superficial layer of horn can be removed to reveal a second layer of horn developing beneath. It is frequently found secondary to white line abscesses or foreign body penetration.

Clinical features: removal of the under-run sole in 7.27 reveals a thin layer of epidermal horn covering the corium. The detached horn is often called a "false sole." In another example (7.15) the point of the hoof knife is lifting the false sole. In other cases acute coriosis may lead to a total but temporary cessation of horn production, and the production of a secondary or false sole, with no outward signs of penetration or white line disease.

Management: the under-run false sole horn is trimmed off to stimulate regrowth of the underlying horn.

Vertical fissure (vertical sandcrack)

Definition: a vertical split, of varying depth, in the hoof wall running from the coronary band toward the weight-bearing surface at the sole, more common in heavy beef breeds.

Clinical features: vertical fissures occur as a result of damage to the superficial periople and underlying coronary band, e.g., following hot, dry weather, or damage to the coronary band from trauma or a digital dermatitis infection. Both claws of the overgrown left forefoot in 7.29 are affected, although the major fissure appears only on the medial claw. Note its irregular course and its origin at the coronary band (A). Note also the section (B), which is slightly loose due to an oblique crack at (C). In 7.30 an extensive, wide, vertical horn crack is shown, in which the laminae are very liable to become exposed, resulting in severe lameness, even though little pus may be present. Another beef cow presented as acutely lame, and extensive paring of a vertical fissure in the front foot eventually led to the release of pus (7.31) and resolution

7.29. Bilateral (lateral and medial) vertical horn fissures in Angus bull

7.32. Vertical fissure with granulation tissue protruding

of the lameness. In advanced cases (7.32), where granulation tissue protrudes from the fissure, it is highly probable that an inflamed corium has produced a proliferative osteitis of the extensor process of the pedal bone, and the expanded bone will no longer fit inside the confined space of the hoof.

Management: the fissure should be opened with a hoof knife and under-run or weightbearing horn on each side of the crack removed, as should any hinged portion of horn, thus reducing the movement of the fissure. If granulation tissue is protruding from the fissure, as in 7.32, it is likely that there is also an osteomyelitis of the pedal bone. Digit amputation is then the only treatment. Supplementary biotin has been shown to decrease the prevalence in beef cattle. Control in dairy herds necessitates lowering the incidence of digital dermatitis.

Horizontal fissure (horizontal sandcrack)

7.30. Vertical horn crack

Definition: horizontal fissures result from a temporary cessation of horn formation, often as a result of severe illness or a metabolic disturbance. If the cessation was marked, the fissure may extend down to the corium. Less severe disruptions cause simple lines of interrupted horn growth, sometimes known as "hardship lines." Unlike vertical fissures, these are usually evident in all eight claws.

Clinical features: in 7.33 both claws are affected: the handheld, cracked, medial hoof wall resulted from a temporary cessation of horn formation 4 months previously, following an abrupt dietary change. Because the length of the anterior wall is greater than the height of the heel, the "thimble" of horn eventually loses its support from the heel, but remains attached at the toe. Lameness results from the pressure of the hinged portion of horn on the underlying laminae, or from exposure of the sensitive laminae when the thimble becomes detached ("broken toe"). In 7.33 a smaller fissure of the lateral claw has been partially trimmed off, without exposing sensitive laminae, to reduce movement of the thimble.

7.31. Vertical fissure

7.33. Horizontal fissure (or sandcrack) in both claws

Sometimes both claws of all four feet may be affected as a result of a severe systemic insult, e.g., following acute mastitis, foot-and-mouth disease, or acute metritis.

Management: herds with a high incidence of horizontal fissures must be suffering periodic bouts of coriosis/laminitis, the cause of which needs identification and correction. Dietary factors and/or disease could be involved, especially in the periparturient cow. Investigation of a herd problem begins with a detailed examination of the history of the transition cow.

Corkscrew claw

Definition: the claw, usually the lateral claw of both hind legs, is twisted spirally throughout its length.

Clinical features: the lateral claw of the front or the hind feet can be affected by this partially heritable growth defect. The overgrown lateral toe in 7.34 deviates upward, and in the same digit, the abaxial wall curls under the sole (7.35), inevitably altering the weightbearing surfaces. The axial sole overgrowth (A) consequently becomes a major weightbearing surface and lameness can

7.35. Same digit as 7.34: abaxial lateral claw wall curls under sole

result from sole ulcers and/or pedal bone compression (see also 7.11). In the pedal bone specimen in 7.36, osteolysis secondary to corkscrew claw compression is seen near the toe, at A. The left pedal bone and the cavitation are normal. 7.35 also shows early bilateral heel erosion (see also 7.67), and cavitation of the sole of the medial claw due to impaction by debris.

Scissor claw

Definition: scissor claw differs from corkscrew claw in that one toe grows across the other, there is less wall involvement, and rotation along a longitudinal axis is absent.

Clinical features: in 7.37 the wall of the left claw curls slightly axially at the point of contact with the ground, and may form a false sole. Slight mechanical lameness can result from the pressure of one toe on top of the other during walking.

Management: both corkscrew claw and scissor claw require repeated radical trimming. Intensive farming practice usually necessitates early culling for economic reasons.

7.34. Corkscrew claw: lateral claw

7.36. Pedal bone specimen showing osteolysis at toe (A) (Japan)

7.37.   Scissor claw with lateral claw curling axially

Complications of digital hoof disorders

Superficial under-running of the corium is easily treated by removal of separated horn and allowing regrowth of new hoof. Infection of deeper tissues leads to additional clinical signs especially swelling around the coronary band of the affected digit, and usually a more severe and protracted lameness. A range of conditions may be seen including abscesses at the coronary band or the heel, rupture of the deep flexor tendon, and deeper sepsis.

Abscess at the coronary band

Infection originating at the white line has passed proximally under the hoof wall to the coronet in 7.38, where it has penetrated the deeper tissues of the collateral digital ligaments to produce a septic cellulitis, with pronounced swelling around the coronary band. As well as highlighting the overgrowth of the sole horn, this chronic lesion shows that the horn wall is detached from the coronet beneath the abscess. The affected toe has deviated dorsally, suggesting partial rupture of the flexor tendon, and leading to relative horn overgrowth from lack of wear.

7.38.   Abscess at coronary band with septic cellulitis

7.39.   Abscess at heel (retroarticular): digital cushion (A)

Management: remove all under run horn to expose the infection tracking dorsally over the laminar and then papillary corium, and drain any deeper abscesses. Aggressive parenteral antibiotics for at least 1 week.

Abscess at heel (retroarticular abscess; septic navicular bursitis)

Definition: an abscess in the synovial space between the deep flexor tendon and the navicular bone, usually a consequence of neglected or infected sole ulcers.

Clinical features: severe lameness and swelling of the heel area and coronary band, which may extend dorsally toward the fetlock and above. In a longitudinal section of a claw (7.39), purulent infection can be seen in the digital cushion (A) adjacent to the navicular bone, the deep digital flexor tendon (B), and adjacent to the pedal joint (C). This is sometimes referred to as a retroarticular abscess, and needs surgical drainage. Similarly 7.40 shows heel enlargement and a purulent exudate, probably from an infected navicular bursa or a retroarticular

7.40.   Massive heel enlargement due to infected navicular bursa or retroarticular abscess

7.41. Ruptured deep flexor tendon and plantigrade toe

abscess discharging through the original ulcer site (A). A wooden block has been applied to the sound claw. Flexor tendon rupture (7.42) may result from complicated cases (see below).

Management: removal of all under-run horn, drainage of abscesses, usually through the original sole ulcer site, by curettage and repeated flushing over several days, and aggressive antibiotic therapy. Distal joint sepsis requires amputation or joint fusion, but many cases are best culled on welfare and economic grounds.

Rupture of the deep flexor tendon

Clinical features: complications from severe white line abscess, sole ulcer, or, as in 7.41, retroarticular heel abscess can lead to infection and the subsequent rupture of the deep flexor tendon. In 7.41 the coronary band is severely distorted, the heel is swollen, and the toe deviates upward (plantigrade), leading to continual overgrowth and lack of wear of the affected claw. A longitudinal section of a septic digit (7.42) reveals the site of an ulcer

that perforated the sole horn (A), and the point of rupture of the deep flexor tendon (B). Note the horn overgrowth at the toe. At this stage the joint is not affected and recovery is possible with prompt treatment.

Management: prompt drainage of any abscess in the acute phase. Regular trimming of the upturned and overgrown toe in the longer term. Many cases then remain productive for several years.

Septic pedal arthritis (distal interphalangeal sepsis)

Definition: infection of the distal interphalangeal joint (pedal joint).

Clinical features: pedal arthritis typically results from a severe or neglected white line abscess, sole ulcer or interdigital necrobacillosis infection and produces severe, often non-weightbearing, lameness. Note the marked unilateral enlargement of the left heel in 7.43, with inflammation tracking up toward the fetlock and causing distortion of the claw. The navicular bursa and pedal joint are also infected, producing a septic pedal arthritis. Gross enlargement can result in lifting of digital sole and heel horn, especially at the heel and toward the interdigital space. The Hereford cow in 7.44 had been lame for 8 weeks. The affected lateral claw is grossly enlarged and inflamed, there is swelling of the coronet and separation of horn at the coronary band (A), and granulation tissue protrudes into the interdigital space at the point where pus discharges from the infected joint. Despite a less severe degree of swelling in the more

7

7.42. Flexor tendon rupture following retroarticular abscess

7.43. Septic pedal arthritis following deep infection

7.44. Septic pedal arthritis with horn separation at coronet and interdigital granulation in cow (Hereford)

7.45. Septic pedal arthritis with hoof avulsion from septic coronitis

chronic case in 7.45, the hoof on the affected lateral claw is being avulsed by pressure and necrosis from a septic coronitis.

Long-standing digital infections may lead to an osteitis and a proliferation of new bone, as in 7.46, which is a boiled-out specimen of a chronically infected sole ulcer in a Holstein cow. A deep cavity was present at the ulcer site, with extensive new bone proliferation in the navicular bone, digital cushion, and coronary areas. When P1, P2, and P3 became ankylosed, the severity of lameness decreased. In 7.47, which is a sagittal section following digital amputation, necrosis in the navicular bone has extended to cause severe sepsis in the distal joint. Infection at the coronary band (B) has produced swelling above the coronet.

Management: when septic pedal arthritis has been confirmed, early digit amputation to prevent further complications is often the best option, but some cases are best culled on welfare and economic grounds. Removal of all under-run horn, deep pedal curettage, flushing, and aggressive antibiotic therapy may prove effective. Insertion of a drainage tube along the track of the original

discharging fistula to exit above the coronary band is easily achieved and improves drainage. Cases involving a marked bony swelling above the coronary band from extensive and longer-term periostitis may achieve joint ankylosis, and then continue a productive life.

Disorders of the digital skin and heels

Whereas hoof disorders arise from the corium and are largely managemental in origin, diseases of the interdigital skin have a large infectious component.

Interdigital necrobacillosis (phlegmona interdigitalis, "foul", "footrot")

Definition: a common cause of lameness, interdigital necrobacillosis is an infection of the dermal layers of interdigital skin associated with *Fusobacterium necrophorum* and other bacteria such as *Porphyromonas assacharolytica* and *Prevotella* spp. Infection starts in the dermis.

7.46. Bone specimen of osteitis secondary to joint sepsis

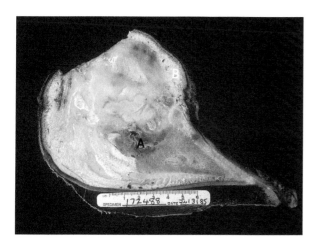

7.47. Sagittal section of claw with septic pedal arthritis

7.49. Interdigital necrobacillosis: exposure of deeper dermis

Clinical features: early cases have an obvious lameness and show a symmetrical, bilateral, hyperemic swelling of the heel bulbs that may extend to the accessory digits. At this stage, the interdigital skin is swollen but intact, and the claws appear to be pushed apart when the animal stands. After 24–48 hours the interdigital skin splits (7.48) (some sloughed epidermis has been removed), and in later cases the dermis is exposed (7.49). More extensive exposure of the dermis is often seen (7.50), with development of granulation tissue. A foulsmelling, caseous exudate may be present (7.51). 7.52 is a dorsal view of a neglected case after cleansing, with sloughed necrotic debris in the interdigital space. The depth of the necrotic process has caused proliferation of granulation tissue. Early separation of the axial wall of the left claw (A) and swelling of the coronet suggest early inflammatory changes in the pedal joint. The horizontal groove (B) distal to the coronary band indicates that the problem has existed for about 1 month.

A peracute form of interdigital necrobacillosis exists known as "super foul" (7.53), where severe necrosis

7.50. Interdigital necrobacillosis: more extensive exposure of dermis

extends from the interdigital cleft onto the heel skin. The dermal necrosis is savage in onset and there may be joint involvement within 48 hours of initial clinical signs. The same causative organisms are involved, although the antibiotic sensitivity pattern may differ. Prompt and aggressive therapy is vital.

7.48. Interdigital necrobacillosis ("foul", "footrot") with typical skin split

7.51. Interdigital necrobacillosis: caseous exudate and interdigital slough

7

7.52. Neglected case of interdigital necrobacillosis with sloughed debris

Differential diagnosis: interdigital dermatitis (7.65), interdigital foreign body (7.69), digital dermatitis (7.57–7.59).

Management: improved foot hygiene by cleaner floor areas and especially regular (e.g., daily) disinfectant foot bathing can dramatically reduce the incidence. Avoid rough gateways and other surfaces that can traumatize the interdigital cleft. Treatment by parenteral and topical antibiotics is normally successful, although aggressive therapy combined with NSAIDs will be required in herds with "super foul."

Interdigital skin hyperplasia (fibroma, "corn")

Definition: hyperplasia in the interdigital space develops from skin folds adjacent to the axial hoof wall, as shown in 7.54.

7.53. "Super foul", peracute interdigital necrobacillosis with massive necrosis

7.54. Interdigital skin hyperplasia ("fibroma", "corn")

Clinical features: the lesion, which in some cases may be inherited and is then usually bilateral, is a problem in heavier breeds of beef and dairy cows as well as mature beef bulls. Lameness is produced either when the claws pinch the interdigital skin during walking, or following secondary (necrobacillary) infection in areas of pressure necrosis (7.55) and commonly as a result of secondary infection with digital dermatitis. Note the superficial but severe slough of necrotic material. In a few cases hyperplasia is restricted more to the dorsal interdigital space (7.56), when lameness is less likely.

Differential diagnosis: interdigital necrobacillosis (7.48), digital dermatitis (7.57–7.59).

Management: predisposing factors that should be avoided in the control of the condition include irritation to the interdigital skin from trauma; excess stretching of the interdigital skin when walking over rough surfaces; inappropriate claw trimming where the axial wall is removed, the claws splay apart, and the interdigital space is stretched; and chronic irritation from digital dermatitis and interdigital necrobacillosis. Small lesions can be treated by removing overgrowth of the axial wall to minimize pinching, or by regular foot bathing through

7.55. Interdigital skin hyperplasia with secondary infection from pressure necrosis

7.56.   Interdigital skin hyperplasia restricted to dorsal part of space

astringents such as formalin or copper sulfate solutions. Larger lesions require amputation.

Digital dermatitis ("hairy warts", "Mortellaro")

Definition: a bacterial (treponeme) infection of the epidermis of the digital skin. Three species of treponemes are thought to be involved.

Clinical features: the lesion is typically seen on the skin above the heel bulbs, proximal to the interdigital space. On initial inspection, early cases (7.57) show hairs that are erect and matted with a serous exudate. Cleaning off superficial debris (7.58) in a similar case reveals a circular reddened area of epidermitis, 1–2 cm in diameter, with a characteristic stippled "strawberry" appearance, and a pronounced pungent odor. Many cases are first

7.57.   Digital dermatitis in typical site in skin above heels, with erect hairs and mucoid exudate

7.58.   Digital dermatitis with discrete area of epidermitis

7.59.   Advanced digital dermatitis with extensive raw epidermitis and under-run heel horn (Italy)

diagnosed by the odor alone. Affected animals are acutely lame, and very sensitive to touch, even though dermal tissues are not significantly involved (compare interdigital necrobacillosis, 7.48). In advanced lesions (7.59) the heel horn becomes eroded and under-run, with an extensive raw area of epidermitis extending up toward the accessory digits. Although the majority of cases occur at the plantar aspect, ulcerating dorsal lesions (7.60) are not

7.60.   Digital dermatitis: ulcerating dorsal lesion (Netherlands)

7.61. Under-run sole extruding from initial heel lesion of digital dermatitis

7.63. Digital dermatitis "hairy warts"

7

uncommon. Such lesions, involving perioplic horn of the coronary band, may produce complications such as vertical fissure and pedal osteitis, and a much more protracted lameness. Another complication involves an under-run sole from an initial heel lesion (7.61). Many chronic non healing white line lesions and sole ulcers are secondarily infected with digital dermatitis and have the characteristic pungent odor. Beneath these lesions the plantar surface of the pedal bone often develops sharp spicules or exostoses which damage the corium and inhibits healing. Chronic neglected dermatitis lesions produce "hairy warts," seen typically as tufts of proliferating skin at the back of the heel (7.62). A less severe form, where the lesion is dry, is seen in Fig 7.63. Many herds have small 5–25 mm tufts of dry hyperkeratinized skin at the interdigital cleft thought to represent the "carrier" state of digital dermatitis.

Differential diagnosis: interdigital necrobacillosis (7.48), interdigital dermatitis (7.65), mud fever (7.66), heel erosion or slurry heel (7.67).

Management: digital dermatitis is associated with repeated exposure to slurry, especially to the mixture of urine and feces which is typically associated with automated slurry scrapers. Low-grade lesions in dry cows which often rapidly progress to produce raw, open lesions in early lactation can spread infection to other animals in the herd, hence disease is most commonly seen in early to peak lactation. Control is based on improved environmental foot hygiene and regular (e.g., daily) disinfectant foot bathing to prevent lesion development. Antibiotic foot baths may be indicated in herds with a high incidence of open lesions, but are not permitted in some countries. A range of disinfectant foot bath products are used for prevention. Formalin may be the cheapest but its use may be forbidden in some countries, and if used inappropriately it may lead to skin burn (7.64).

More advanced lesions causing lameness can be treated individually by topical antibiotic spray or antibiotics held in place by a dressing. Occasionally surgical removal of large "hairy warts" is required.

Formalin skin burn

Definition: a slough of the superficial epidermal layers associated with inappropriate use of formalin foot baths. This includes prolonged exposure to baths above 5% formaldehyde.

Clinical features: seen especially during hot, dry weather when the digital skin is dry and may absorb

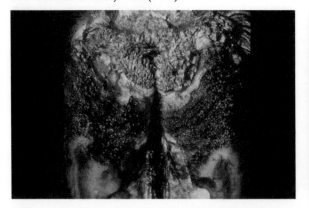

7.62. Typical "hairy warts" in chronic digital dermatitis

7.64. Formalin burn

formalin. Note the thickening of the skin around the coronary band in 7.64, which will feel hard and dry, and has lost its pliability. An area of superficial slough of dead dry skin exposes a raw epidermis beneath. Removal of formalin exposure results in rapid and uncomplicated healing. Fumes emitted from high-concentration baths in hot weather often make cows reluctant to enter.

Differential diagnosis: digital dermatitis (7.57), mud fever (7.66), cutaneous dermatophilosis (3.38, 3.43), photosensitization (3.5–3.9).

Interdigital dermatitis

Interdigital dermatitis is a superficial, moist inflammation of the interdigital epidermis (7.65) not involving the deeper tissues, and hence differs from necrobacillosis (7.48). *Dichelobacter nodosus* has occasionally been recovered from lesions. Several cattle may be affected at one time. Despite the superficial nature of the lesion, lameness is sometimes pronounced. Many consider this lesion to be indistinguishable from digital dermatitis.

Differential diagnosis: interdigital necrobacillosis (7.48), digital dermatitis (7.57–7.59).

Management: topical antibiotic aerosol.

"Mud fever"

Clinical features: mud fever occurs following exposure to cold, wet, muddy conditions and may involve secondary *Dermatophilus* infection (see 3.38). In 7.66 the leg is swollen, especially around the pastern. Lameness was pronounced. The cleansed skin is thickened with a dry eczema and there is some hair loss from the coronet, extending to above the fetlock. Often the dry skin cracks,

7.66. "Mud fever" with thickened dry eczematous skin

leading to areas of superficial hemorrhage. All four limbs may be affected.

Differential diagnosis: digital dermatitis (7.57), formalin burn (7.64), cutaneous dermatophilosis (3.37, 3.42), photosensitization (3.5–3.9).

Management: affected areas should be thoroughly washed and a greasy antiseptic ointment rubbed onto the area. Alternatively the skin may be sprayed with high emollient teat dip. Severe cases benefit from a 3-day course of systemic penicillin.

Heel erosion ("slurry heel")

Definition: erosion of the heel horn. The heel is an important weightbearing surface. Its normal structure has been demonstrated in preceding illustrations, e.g., 7.55.

Clinical features: erosion is commonly seen in housed dairy cows that stand in slurry. Loss of the heel horn destabilizes the hoof, alters weightbearing, increases concussion, and by a caudoventral rotation of the pedal bone may predispose to sole ulcers. Slurry heel may be related to digital and interdigital dermatitis. *Bacteroides nodosus* has occasionally been isolated from both lesions. In 7.67 the original smooth horn has been eroded, producing a deep fissure in the left heel. More severe erosion of the right (lateral) heel horn has led to the appearance

7.65. Interdigital dermatitis with superficial moist inflammation

7.67. Heel erosion ("slurry heel") with heel horn erosion, and deep heel fissure

7.68. Severe heel erosion and digital dermatitis

of granulation tissue from the sole. In the advanced case of 7.68 both heels are almost completely eroded. Digital dermatitis and slurry heel often occur together, as in 7.68, as poor environmental hygiene predisposes to both conditions.

Differential diagnosis: digital dermatitis (7.57).

Management: frequent disinfectant foot bathing reduces the incidence in housed cattle, and spontaneous recovery is seen when cattle are kept at pasture. Some cases require trimming to remove flaps of horn that trap debris, but care is needed, otherwise excess removal of heel horn will lead to caudal ventral rotation of the claw, thus predisposing to sole ulcers.

Interdigital foreign body

Clinical features: in 7.69 a stone is impacted in the interdigital space, ulcerating the axial skin of the left claw.

Small pieces of twig, especially thorns, can lie longitudinally in the cleft, damaging the interdigital skin and leading to secondary necrobacillosis (see also 7.28).

Differential diagnosis: interdigital necrobacillosis.

Management: removal and careful examination of the depth and extent of interdigital trauma. Topical antibiotic.

Fracture of the distal phalanx

Definition: occurring primarily in the front feet, distal phalangeal fracture is usually traumatic and intra-articular, although it may be pathologically associated with fluorosis (13.31) or osteomyelitis.

Clinical features: the medial claw is often involved, forcing the animal to adopt a crosslegged stance, and hence transferring weight to the lateral claw (7.70). The fracture line (A) in 7.71 runs vertically from the distal interphalangeal (pedal) joint, and the two fragments of pedal bone are separated. This type of fracture leads to a sudden onset of severe lameness, often with no initial visible signs of heat or swelling. Later, the affected claw may be palpably hotter, but in the early stages diagnosis without radiography is difficult. The most common cause of a crossed foreleg stance is however bilateral sole ulceration.

Differential diagnosis: bilateral ulcers of medial claws of forefeet, foreign body perforation of the interdigital space or the sole.

Management: as the bone is "self-splinted" by the hoof casing, most cases recover with limited intervention.

7.69. Interdigital foreign body (stone)

7.70. Stance in fracture of medial distal phalanx of left foreleg

7.71. Radiograph of distal limb with intra-articular fracture line (A)

7.72. Acute coriosis: abducted forelegs, arched back, hind limbs forward (USA)

A surgical block put on the sound claw minimizes weight-bearing on the affected claw, improving the welfare of the cow by abolition of pain, and speeding the healing process.

Laminitis

Definition: although "laminitis" remains a widely used term, rarely are changes limited to the laminar area of the corium, which opposes ventral areas of the axial and abaxial hoof wall only. The dorsal areas and corium covering the sole are papillary corium (i.e., where the horn is produced), hence hemorrhage on the sole cannot be laminitis, as laminae are absent there. In most instances inflammation of the entire corium is involved, hence the term "coriosis" is more appropriate. Recent research into the pathogenesis of sole ulcers and white line disease has suggested that the laminar corium remains normal (i.e., there is no inflammatory process present) when the distal phalanx sinks, hence use of the term laminitis may not be justified in cattle. The primary changes are microvascular, the causes being multifactorial and include trauma, periparturient changes, infections, metabolic disease, and dietary disturbances.

Acute coriosis, laminitis and sole hemorrhage

Clinical features: the Friesian cow in 7.72 has a typical acute laminitic stance: the front legs are abducted, the hind legs are placed forward under the abdomen, the back is arched, the neck is extended, the head is held low, and the tail is slightly raised. Hoof changes following laminitis/coriosis are shown in 7.73. Hemorrhage can be seen over the heel bulb and along the white line. Note the black debris impacted into the widened white line towards the heel, which could result in white line infection (7.6). Intense congestion of the blood vessels in the corium is the most probable cause of the blood

clot in the sole horn at the toe. The heifer had calved 2 months previously and the coriosis/laminitis was probably the result of depressed horn synthesis around the time of calving, leading to a thin sole susceptible to bruising, and a change from a fibrous to a high-concentrate diet (producing acidosis), combined with excessive standing on concrete. The condition is frequently seen when heifers that have been reared in yards or on pasture are introduced postpartum into cubicles for the first time.

The gross widening and hemorrhage of the white line in the 3-year-old Simmental bull (7.74) was the result of excessive exercise in a cubicle-housed dairy herd over several months, at the beginning of which acute laminitis developed. These changes caused softening of the white line, which then permitted penetration of dirt, and finally resulted in acute lameness due to the under-run sole. White line abscesses (7.6–7.9) and sole ulcers (7.13–7.16) are the common sequel to acute coriosis.

7.73. Acute coriosis: hoof changes include hemorrhage along white line and at heel

7

7.74.   Chronic coriosis with widened and hemorrhagic white line (Simmental bull, 3 years old)

Chronic coriosis, laminitis

Clinical features: in this longitudinal section (7.75) through the foot of a 6-year-old Shorthorn bull with early chronic coriosis/laminitis, the sole laminae are thickened and hemorrhagic, and pink striations indicate that there is blood in the sole horn, particularly at the toe. The pedal bone is displaced downwards, away from the overlying hoof wall. At a later stage (7.76), the line of hemorrhage (A) in the sole horn beneath the pedal bone is easily recognizable. The inflammatory insult responsible for this line would have occurred about 5 weeks previously. Note the thickening and the dorsal deviation of the toe. These changes lead to growth irregularities of the type seen in 7.77 and 7.78. In 7.77 the wall of the outer claw (left) is curling axially. A deep heel fissure and an obvious false sole are developing. The medial claw (right) has an expanded white line. Both hind claws in 7.78 are elongated and the heels are sunken. The toe angle is small, there are prominent horizontal lines, and the periople at the coronary band is flaky.

Management: the causes and control of coriosis have been discussed under sections on white line disorders, sole ulcers, and horizontal fissures.

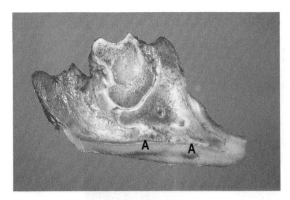

7.76.   Chronic coriosis (autopsy) with sole hemorrhage and dorsal deviation of toe

7.77.   Chronic coriosis with irregular growth, deep heel fissure, and false sole

7.75.   Chronic coroisis (autopsy) with thick solar laminae and pink striations (Shorthorn bull, 6 years old)

7.78.   Chronic coriosis laminitis, elongated claws with horizontal rings

Upper limb and spine

Introduction

The illustrations in this section have been grouped primarily by affected area and type of damage. Although the "downer cow" syndrome is not a physical injury, it is included here because many of the conditions subsequently illustrated can be a consequence of the "downer cow." This is followed by spinal conditions, and trauma affecting joints and long bones (e.g., fractures). Paralyses, excluding those illustrated in the downer cow section, form another small group. Infectious causes are pictured in the septic arthritides section. Finally, a miscellaneous group includes vitamin and mineral deficiencies and metabolic disorders that can result in lameness.

Downer cow

Definition: animals that fail to rise after treatment for hypocalcemia, (p. 161; see 9.6, 9.7) and where no obvious cause of recumbency can be diagnosed, are commonly referred to as "downer" cows. The reason often remains obscure.

Clinical features: metabolic disease, and specifically a nonresponsive milk fever or hypocalcemia (see 9.6, 9.7), is the major cause of the downer cow syndrome. Such cows fail to rise after treatment for hypocalcemia. The etiology is often puzzling. Lying on hard concrete or on the edge of the gutter in a standing or cubicle for as little as 6 hours can cause permanent nerve damage in the hind leg. Struggling may cause dislocation of the hip joint, muscle rupture, femoral fracture, or other trauma that prevents the animal from rising, despite being normocalcemic. Other more insidious conditions, such as metritis, mastitis, and toxicities, can also cause a cow or a bull to become a downer. Blood changes include a rapid elevation of muscle enzymes, such as serum glutamic-oxaloacetic transaminase (SGOT) and creatine phosphokinase (CPK), as a result of ischemic muscle necrosis.

Differential diagnosis: hypocalcemia with magnesium or phosphorus deficiency, femoral or tibial fracture (7.89, 7.112), spinal trauma (7.94), peroneal or sciatic paralysis, hip luxation (7.86, 7.87), acute mastitis, metritis, coccygeal fracture.

Management: care of the downer cow is very important. Good nursing on a soft surface, e.g., straw on top of sand, which provides an adequate grip when the animal attempts to rise, is the prime requirement. Unless she is rolling from side to side herself, she should be turned at least once and preferably several times daily. Loss of appetite, progressive signs of dullness, inability to sit up

7.79. Compartment syndrome with pronounced gluteal swelling

7.80. Spinal or pelvic damage: "dog sitting position" or posterior paresis in cow (Simmental)

unaided, and toxicity suggest a poor prognosis, but some alert downers have been known to rise spontaneously after several weeks. Hip clamps, slings, and inflatable bags have a role in temporarily elevating the hindquarters.

Compartment syndrome

Definition: ischemic muscle degeneration of the hind limb leading to intense pain, limb dysfunction, and eventual toxemia from byproducts of muscle breakdown.

Clinical features: the cow in 7.79 had been recumbent on her right side for 24 hours, and was turned over to help examination of the right leg. There was pronounced swelling and thickening of the gluteal region and further swelling around the tibia. On palpation the enlargement was hard and painful. The prognosis for such cases is poor. The animal is disinclined to move and the resulting toxemia leads to anorexia.

Differential diagnosis: primary nerve paralysis (7.142–7.144), pelvic fracture (7.109, 7.110), femoral fracture (7.89).

Management: put on soft bedding, turn from side to side several times daily, and ensure access to feed and water.

Spinal or pelvic damage

Clinical features: suddenly, after dystocia, the mature Simmental female in 7.80 adopted this "dog-sitting" position, which is suggestive of lumbar or pelvic canal trauma. The posterior paresis resolved after 3 weeks, and the cow recovered completely. Occasionally, this odd position is habitual as a result of spondylarthrosis. Progressively severe posterior paresis with "knuckling" of the hind fetlocks (7.81) developed in this mature Holstein cow as a result of vertebral lymphoma. Autopsy of a similar case (7.82) shows a transverse section of the caudal lumbar vertebral area with yellow-brown lymphomatous tissue

7.81. Progressive posterior paresis due to spinal lymphoma in cow (Holstein) (USA)

(A) and normal, white, epidural fat within the spinal canal. The lymphoma caused marked compression of the spinal nerves, including the sciatic supply. Lymphosarcomatous tissue (yellow) is seen to be infiltrating the bodies of several lumbar vertebrae (7.83), causing progressive posterior paresis.

7.82. Lymphoma in lumbar spinal canal (A) at autopsy

7.83. Lymphomatous infiltration of bodies of several lumbar spinal vertebrae (yellow)

7.84. Lumbar spondylosis in cow

The Friesian cow in 7.84 had lumbar spondylosis, and stood and walked only with great difficulty. Body condition is very poor and the thoracolumbar spine is convex and prominent owing to muscle atrophy. The position of the hind legs relieves pain on spinal nerves. A lateral radiograph of a similar case (7.85) shows lumbar degenerative arthropathy, with ventral osteophyte proliferation (A). Progressive ankylosis brings a risk of fracture of the newly deposited bone of the spinal body, leading to the downer syndrome.

Differential diagnosis: metabolic disease or toxic infection, hind limb trauma (7.86–7.93).

Management: some cases (7.80) respond to good nursing in a deeply bedded loose box. Any deterioration necessitates an immediate full clinical re-examination.

Dislocated hip

Clinical features: although hip dislocation can be a cause of a "downer cow", it is more commonly a consequence of injury from falling, e.g., during estrus activity. Craniodorsal dislocations are more frequent (80% of hip dislocations), as in the cow in 7.86, which shows an abnormal posture and silhouette of the left leg. In the Friesian heifer in 7.87 the left femoral head is dislocated upward and forward (craniodorsally). The bony landmarks of the hindquarters are incongruent. The left gluteal musculature is prominent owing to dorsal displacement of the greater femoral trochanter (A). Crepitus can occasionally be detected on circumrotation of the femur. Ventral (7.88, a crossbred Charolais cow which jumped off a bank down into a roadway) and caudal dislocation of the femoral head into the obturator foramen may also occur, when damage may be caused to the obturator nerve (7.91). In 7.88 the femoral greater trochanter is displaced ventrally from its usual location.

Differential diagnosis: pelvic fracture (7.110), proximal femoral fracture (7.89, 7.90, 7.112), obturator paralysis (7.91, 7.92), spinal fracture (7.94, 7.95).

Management: early cases may be reduced by manipulation, especially in younger cattle with craniodorsal luxation. Dislocations incurred over 24 hours previously are usually culled as untreatable.

Fractured femur

Clinical features: most femoral fractures in periparturient animals occur close to the femoral head and are diagnosed on the basis of abnormal limb position and the detection of crepitus on limb movement. The downer cow in 7.89 has a right femoral midshaft fracture and related soft-tissue swelling. The lower part of the right

7.85. Lateral radiograph of lumbar spine with severe degenerative arthropathy and ventral osteophytes (A)

7

7.86. Craniodorsal hip dislocation (left) with obvious asymmetry

limb is deviated laterally owing to outward movement of the lower femoral shaft. The area is very painful. Such fractures do not always result in recumbency. Another femoral fracture (7.90) shows extensive soft tissue swelling and the forward and outward position of the leg. After one or two attempts, cattle usually abandon further efforts to stand. The underlying, nonfractured hind leg is liable to develop severe ischemic muscle necrosis (see p. 122). Femoral fracture in calves is discussed and shown in 7.112.

Differential diagnosis: dislocated hip (7.86, 7.87), pelvic fracture (7.109, 7.110).

Management: usually untreatable except for mid or distal shaft fractures in immature cattle where internal fixation (plate, pins) may be attempted in valuable stock.

7.88. Ventral hip dislocation in cow (Charolais crossbred)

Obturator paralysis

Definition: the obturator nerve supplies the adductor muscles of the hind limb. Dystocia from fetal oversize may produce unilateral or bilateral nerve paralysis, with subsequent limb abduction.

Clinical features: in 7.91 the abducted and symmetrical position of the hind legs is characteristic of bilateral obturator paralysis. Less severe cases will simply walk

7.87. Left dorsocranial hip dislocation (A) in heifer

7.89. Right midshaft femoral fracture in downer cow

7.90. Right femoral shaft fracture in standing cow showing abnormal stance

7.91. Bilateral obturator paralysis in recumbent cow

with limb abduction, but if allowed onto slippery concrete (as happened in 7.91), may slip ("do the splits"), and a dislocated hip or femoral fracture may result as a secondary feature. Compare the degree of limb adduction in 7.91 with that in 7.92, where there is secondary hip or femoral damage. This cow will not recover. Another cow (7.93), partially recovered from an obturator paralysis incurred 9 months previously, still abducts the right leg when walking; the left leg is normal and weightbearing.

7.92. Bilateral obturator paralysis with secondary hip or femoral damage

7.93. Cow 9 months after onset of right obturator paralysis

Differential diagnosis: dislocated hip (7.86, 7.87), femoral fracture (7.89, 7.90).

Management: confinement to a well-bedded straw box. If obturator paralysis is suspected, the animal should be retained on a soft surface where grip is optimal until locomotion has improved. Hobbles applied to the fetlocks or hocks will help to prevent excessive abduction and may permit the cow safely to walk for milking, etc. Regular brief attempts may be made with a hip clamp to raise the cow to a standing position to assess development and to aid the circulation to the hind limbs.

Spinal conditions

Spinal compression fracture

Clinical features: spinal cord compression (A) (7.94) can be caused by a vertebral fracture (B). Posterior paresis had developed suddenly in this 8-month-old Holstein heifer and was probably associated with clinical rickets of several months' duration. A compression fracture had resulted in the vertebral body being slowly forced dorsally, causing kyphosis (arched back). The spinal canal became progressively stenosed and another fracture of the rachitic bone then compressed the spinal cord. Both

7.94. Spinal cord compression involving vertebral fracture in heifer at autopsy (Holstein) (USA)

7.95. Kyphosis due to lumbar trauma

7.97. Scoliosis (kyphosis) in crossbred calf

compression fractures and septic foci in vertebral growth plates usually occur in younger cattle.

In a Friesian steer that suddenly developed kyphosis, with a discretely localized convexity of the caudal thoracic spine (7.95), its rapid deterioration necessitated slaughter. Autopsy examination revealed a collapsed and infected intervertebral disc space (7.96) between the first (A) and second (B) lumbar vertebrae, resulting from a septic physitis. Deviation of the spinal canal and some spinal cord compression were evident (C). Kyphosis can also be congenital, and is progressive with increasing age. Many affected calves eventually become recumbent. Scoliosis and kyphosis are evident in this Friesian crossbred calf (7.97), and such cases, usually progressive, should be culled as unthrifty. Spinal scoliosis of iatrogenic origin is seen in 7.98. A mature Holstein cow, operated for an LDA under left paravertebral analgesia (T13, L1, L2, 3 × 20 mL lidocaine hydrochloride) immediately developed scoliosis (viewed from above), and failed to recover in the succeeding week, necessitating cull. Autopsy was not possible, but unusually, severe damage to the left lumbar spinal cord must be assumed.

Differential diagnosis: other types of spinal trauma, e.g., infiltrating lymphosarcomatous masses, pelvic or sacral fracture, osteomyelitis.

Management: early identification and where possible correction of the primary cause is clearly essential. Most affected animals require slaughter, but it may be possible to prevent further cases by dietary management. High-concentrate maize-based diets with no supplementary minerals are commonly involved, and may also lead to spontaneous limb fractures.

Spinal (vertebral) spondylopathy

Definition: any vertebral disease including osteomyelitis, spinal abscessation, and ankylosis (spondylosis).

Clinical features: osteomyelitis of the spinal vertebrae is a painful progressive disease, seen in both young and mature animals as a result of hematogenous spread. The cow in 7.99 had a pained expression due to vertebral abscessation, walked stiffly and was soon reluctant to stand.

Specimen 7.100 is a longitudinal section of the thoracolumbar spine of a 6-month-old Holstein calf. Osteomyelitis affects the whole depth of a lumbar vertebral physis (growth plate). The intervertebral disc has been destroyed and the vertebral canal is stenosed. Hemorrhage is evident beneath the meninges over the stenosed cord. The infection was probably hematogenous (*Arcanobacterium pyogenes* was isolated).

7.96. Lumbar spine at autopsy of 7.97 with collapsed and infected intervertebral disc (L1–L2)

7.98. Spinal scoliosis of iatrogenic origin, following paravertebral analgesia for LDA surgery (USA) (View from above standing cow)

7.99. Spinal osteomyelitis in Friesian cow (USA)

7.101. Spinal (vertebral) spondylopathy stance in cow (Holstein)

The cow in 7.101 has an arched thoracolumbar spine and the hind feet are placed further to the rear than normal. The right hind foot is lifted in an attempt to relieve spinal pain. Such cows often "paddle" with the hind legs and may have difficulty in rising. The condition (compare lumbar spondylosis (7.84) and spinal osteomyelitis (7.99)), is a slowly progressive, aseptic process. Proliferating bone on the spinal bodies may eventually produce ankylosis (7.85).

Differential diagnosis: spinal osteomyelitis (7.99, 7.100), spinal compression fractures (7.94–7.97).

Management: most cases are slowly or rapidly progressive and should be culled on welfare grounds, especially when rapidly becoming recumbent.

Cervical spinal fracture

A fracture of the fifth and sixth cervical vertebrae made the 2-year-old Friesian heifer in 7.102 unable to lift the

head and neck. A prominent dip is apparent in the dorsal cervical spine, in front of the scapula. In another similar case, the cow grazed on her knees as she was unable to bend her neck sufficiently to reach the pasture.

Sacroiliac subluxation and luxation

Definition: the ligamentous attachment at the junction of the pelvis and the sacrum relaxes in the periparturient animal to allow passage of the fetus through the birth canal. Rotation of the sacrum on the spine can result when severe traction is applied to an oversized fetus. A partial loss of integrity of the fibrous union of the sacroiliac joint (subluxation) occasionally results, as can complete loss of contact of the two articular surfaces (luxation).

Clinical features: subluxation can cause temporary recumbency, the downer cow syndrome (p. 121). The wings of the ilium in the Friesian cow (7.103) are raised relative to the lumbar spine. Rectal palpation revealed the sacral promontory to be pushed backward and depressed, resulting in a reduced dorsoventral diameter of the pelvic

7.100. Osteomyelitis in lumbar growth plate of calf at autopsy (Holstein, 6 months old)

7.102. Cervical (C5–6) fracture in heifer (Friesian, 2 years old)

7.103. Sacroiliac subluxation with raised ilial wings in cow (Friesian) (Belgium)

7.105. Crushed tail head

inlet. In contrast, a cow with a complete luxation (with no persisting contact of the sacrum with the ilial wings) is unlikely to recover to a normal stance and gait.

Differential diagnosis: pelvic fracture (7.109–7.111), lumbar spinal fracture, spinal spondylopathy (7.99, 7.100), downer cow syndrome.

Management: cases of subluxation often improve over a few days to survive the lactation, but cases with complete luxation should be culled as soon as possible. Cows with subluxation should not be retained for breeding as the reduced pelvic inlet could predispose to dystocia.

Sacrococcygeal fracture and tail paralysis

Clinical features: fractures in this region may involve a "crushed or broken tail head" and tail paralysis. 7.104 shows the dorsal pelvic area of a Friesian cow with a sacral fracture and ventral displacement of caudal lumbar spine and sacrum. Note how the prominent tuber ischii protrude well above the tail head. Another form is shown in 7.105, where progressive posterior paresis developed

Constriction of neural canal   **Site of original fracture**

7.106. Crushed tail head and sacral damage, leading to posterior paresis (France)

in a lactating Red Friesian with a crushed tail head and sacral damage. Note the loss in condition. The cow had recently been served by a bull. A loose, flaccid tail with no muscle tone is almost pathognomonic. 7.106 shows a bone specimen of the sacrum of a cow with a similar history to 7.105. The Hereford bull (7.107) could not raise his tail to defecate. The prominent swelling at the

7.104. Sacral fracture

7.107. Sacrococcygeal fracture in bull unable to raise tail (Hereford)

7.108. Sacrococcygeal fracture in heifer (Guernsey, 2 years old)

7.109. Open fracture of left ilial wing in cow with gross contamination

tailhead (A) is an old sacrococcygeal fracture, which resulted from a fall during attempted service of a cow, and led to compression of the coccygeal nerve supply. However, sacrococcygeal fracture does not invariably lead to nerve dysfunction, but sometimes only to minor disfigurement, as in the 2-year-old Guernsey heifer in 7.108. The growing animal is especially susceptible to compression fractures of the spine and to localization of metastatic septic foci in the growth plates of vertebral bodies (compare 7.99, 7.100).

Management: if only the tail is affected, clipping off tail hair reduces fecal contamination of the udder, and many cases eventually recover. "Crushed tail head" is typically seen 1–2 days after estrus, and NSAID therapy should be instigated as soon as clinical signs appear. If cows are knuckled at the fetlock, as in 7.105, they should be housed separately on a nonslip surface. Some are so badly affected that they are no longer safe to be brought in to be milked, whilst severe cases are unable to stand unaided. These latter cases should be culled. Most cases do recover, but it may take several months.

Trauma of joints and long bones

Pelvic fracture

Definition: most pelvic fractures involve the ilial wing and are of minor significance. Iliac shaft and pubic fractures are much less common but cause severe lameness and sometimes recumbency, as in the downer cow.

Clinical features: an open fracture of the left ilial wing of the cow in 7.109 is grossly contaminated, and as drainage is poor, lesions in this area are slow to heal. Such fractures arise from trauma incurred with rough handling or overcrowding, when cows are rushed through doorways, or from a sudden fall onto a hard surface. Most fractures of the ilial wing are closed, the fragment of bone being pulled downward by the fascia lata, as in the

7.110. Closed fracture of right ilial wing in cow ("dropped hip") (Guernsey)

Guernsey cow (7.110), where the bony prominence is absent ("dropped hip") on the right side. In other cases, the skin over the bone becomes gangrenous and sloughs (7.111). Most ilial wing fractures are nothing more than cosmetic blemishes.

Management: routine wound treatment is needed in open cases, after removal of any bone fragments. Resection of protruding bone promotes healing.

7.111. Skin slough over right ilial wing following fracture

7

7.112.   Stance in femoral shaft fracture in calf (Simmental)

Femoral fracture

Clinical features: the soft tissue swelling in this Simmental bull calf (7.112) overlies a femoral shaft fracture of 2 days' duration. The stance could be confused with femoral paralysis, or a hip injury such as coxofemoral luxation or femoral neck fracture. Other femoral fractures are shown in 7.89 and 7.90.

Management: surgical repair is often indicated. Immobilization with a limb cast is not possible. Euthanasia is often carried out on economic and welfare grounds.

Patellar luxation

Definition: upward or lateral, intermittent or permanent displacement of the patella, of uncertain etiology.

Clinical features: the respective clinical signs differ markedly (compare 7.113 and 7.114). The right hind leg of the Holstein heifer in 7.113 was held in maximal extension for a few seconds and was then jerked forward. The patella was temporarily fixed above the femoral trochlea. Diagnosis of upward patellar fixation, made on palpation during locomotion, is confirmed by the

response to medial patellar desmotomy. One specific form of upward luxation and fixation occurs in growing and mature cattle, and is also common among draught animals in the Indian subcontinent. Some forms are inherited.

In contrast, the young Holstein calf (7.114) had a flexed stifle. The patella was easily palpable, and luxated lateral to the femoral trochlea, increasing the total width of the joint. Note the accompanying severe quadriceps femoris atrophy and left hind plantigrade stance. Lateral patellar luxation is generally encountered in calves less than 1 month old.

Differential diagnosis: in upward patellar fixation, spastic paresis (7.148); in lateral patellar luxation, femoral paralysis (7.143).

Management: medial patellar desmotomy in the upward luxation or fixation; medial overlap procedure in lateral luxation though prognosis in later surgery is guarded. Some cases of intermittent upward luxation resolve spontaneously.

Degenerative joint disease (DJD)

Definition: a chronic degeneration of the articular cartilage with thickening of the joint capsule and peripheral osteophyte formation in one or more major joints in older cows and bulls, which may be unable to mount for natural service.

Clinical features: degenerative joint disease (DJD) affects the hip and stifle more frequently than other weightbearing joints. This hip joint of an old Hereford cow (7.115) shows the classical features of DJD: extensive erosion of articular cartilage (A), eburnation of the underlying bone (B), and a thickened joint capsule (C). The presence of blood suggests that a more recent traumatic incident had occurred after the chronic changes became established.

Differential diagnosis: DJD of stifle (see aseptic gonitis (7.116–7.118)), pelvic fracture (7.109–7.111).

7.113.   Right patellar luxation (upward) showing marked extension in heifer (Holstein, USA)

7.114.   Right patellar luxation (lateral) in calf (Holstein, USA)

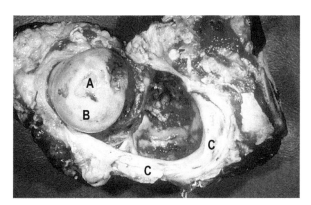

7.115. Degenerative joint disease (DJD) of hip showing erosion, eburnation, and thick joint capsule

Management: rest, confinement, analgesics, and NSAIDs.

Aseptic gonitis (stifle osteoarthritis)

Definition: degenerative joint disease (see DJD on previous page) of one or both stifle joints, often in older cattle.

Clinical features: aseptic or noninfectious gonitis results from trauma, and animals experience a severe and chronic lameness. Some cows have a slow progressive enlargement of the stifle and move the limb without flexing the joint. Muscle atrophy of the limb rapidly develops. The swelling in the yearling Friesian (7.116) comprises fibrosis and inflammatory fluid around the joint with secondary bone proliferation. Typically, young cattle may have a partial rupture of a collateral ligament. Some such cases remain slightly lame owing to a secondary degenerative osteoarthritis. In mature cattle (7.117) cranial cruciate ligament rupture (CrCL) is a common

7.117. Cranial cruciate rupture at autopsy showing chronic changes in stifle joint

cause of severe stifle lameness (ruptured ligament (A)). A lateral radiograph (7.118) of the stifle joint of a similar old beef cow shows considerable cranial movement of the tibial articular surface on the femoral condyles (about 3 cm). A small chip is evident near the tibial eminence (A). The cranial view into the opened stifle joint in 7.117 shows a mere fragment of the CrCL (A), although the caudal cruciate ligament (B) is intact. The medial meniscus is torn and fragmented. The medial femoral condyle shows bone loss from erosion (C), and the margin of the condyle has extensive osteophyte proliferation (D). The palpably thickened joint capsule and bony enlargement are prominent clinical signs of CrCL rupture.

Differential diagnosis: septic gonitis, distal femoral fracture, periarticular abscess.

7.116. Aseptic traumatic gonitis with severe joint swelling in yearling (Friesian)

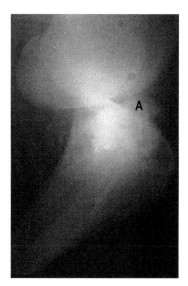

7.118. Lateral radiograph of stifle showing drawer forward position of tibia and bone chip (A)

7.119. Distal metacarpal fracture in calf with severe angulation

Management: few cases will recover. NSAIDs and analgesic drugs may help locomotion, but lactating cows are best confined to yards and loose boxes.

Metacarpal/metatarsal fractures

Definition: fractures of metacarpal/metatarsal shaft may be closed or open. The age range is wide and includes sporadic cases in both young calves and adult cattle.

Clinical features in younger cattle: the Friesian calf in 7.119 had severe angulation following a recent distal metacarpal shaft fracture. The fracture had not been reduced and immobilized. The small amount of overlying soft tissue makes such fractures liable to perforate through the skin and become infected, hence producing osteomyelitis. Such fractures, or separation of the metacarpal physis, are very likely to occur following excessive traction in dystocia. The bilateral metacarpal shaft fractures in the Angus heifer in 7.120 were caused by traction on obstetrical chains placed just above the fetlocks. Note

7.121. Radiograph of metacarpal fracture with epiphyseal separation (Salter type II)

the residual scar. In this view, healing was taking place 2 weeks after external splintage, but note the 10–20° malalignment.

Metacarpal fracture may occur with epiphyseal separation, as seen in the radiograph (7.121). This shows a partial separation and displacement of the distal metacarpal growth plate (A), and fracture of the metaphysis (B) (Salter type II) in a neonatal calf. Metacarpal fracture with epiphyseal separation, is seen in the 8 month old Holstein heifer shown in 7.122. Note the hard, painful swelling on the lateral aspect of the fetlock, and the marked lateral rotation of the limb which could not be realigned.

Differential diagnosis: careful manipulation should reveal whether the shaft is fractured or the distal physis is separated. Radiography can confirm the precise conformation.

7.120. Bilateral metacarpal fracture following excessive traction on chains placed above fetlocks (USA)

7.122. Distal metacarpal epiphyseal fracture

7.123. Metatarsal fracture with two discharging sinuses related to sequestrum

7.124. Septic carpitis and pressure necrosis in heifer (Holstein, 4 months old) (USA)

Management: the prognosis for closed cases is good with careful management such as external support, although the leg may remain malaligned following epiphyseal fracture. Check carefully whether the fracture is open and therefore infected. Such cases, carrying a more guarded prognosis, need debridement and irrigation before external fixation is applied, and an optional "porthole" may be left for catheter and further irrigation. External support (e.g., resin) should extend proximal to the carpus and distal to the coronet. Systemic antibiotics should be given for 5–7 days.

Clinical features in adult cattle: most cases present as a sudden onset lameness. Typical metatarsal/metacarpal shaft fractures are very common and account for 50% of all long bone fractures in adults.

A second type (chip fracture), involving a sequestrum chip from the cortex, is also occasionally seen (7.123) although changes in the metacarpal/metatarsal shafts may be difficult to detect in the early stages. As the condition progresses, a pronounced hard swelling develops, as in 7.123, where two discharging sinuses are visible on the lateral aspect of the left metatarsus. This animal injured her leg as a heifer when transported to the farm several months previously. On X-ray a large saucer-shaped sequestrum of bone cortex was evident on the lateral aspect of the midshaft region of the metatarsus. Most cases are traumatic in origin and the discharge is a foreign body reaction, although bacterial infection may also occur.

Management: the common fracture type should be managed as for calves though the risk of an open fracture is greater. In chip fractures surgical removal of the sequestrum is possible but not easy. In many cases lameness will resolve if exercise is limited for 2–3 months, and although the leg swelling persists this does not cause a problem.

Infectious arthritis (septic arthritis and epiphysitis)

Clinical features: this section excludes joint ill and polyarthritis of calfhood (see 2.48). The usual age range for septic arthritis in calves is 1–3 months. Most forms of septic or infectious arthritis are bacterial in origin. They originate from penetrating wounds, extension from adjacent tissues (both forms being common in digital sepsis, see p. 111), or spread by the hematogenous route. Some examples are given.

In a case of septic carpitis, pressure necrosis of the skin over the carpus (knee) in a 4-month-old Holstein heifer (7.124) has exposed the carpal bones. Note the peripheral epithelialization and necrosis. A lateral radiograph of the flexed carpus (7.125) shows soft tissue

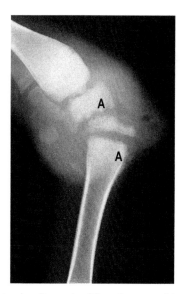

7.125. Lateral radiograph of flexed carpus with severe bone destruction (A)

7.126. Septic carpitis (vertical section) in autopsy specimen (USA)

7.128. Severe sepsis in fetlock joint at autopsy of cow

swelling, bone destruction of the middle and distal rows of carpal bones, and an extensive osseous proliferative reaction (A). A sagittal section through the limb (7.126) confirms the massive tissue destruction. Infection also extends along the tendon sheaths. Detected some weeks earlier such an infection could have been successfully managed.

The 4-month-old calf in 7.127 has a wound (not visible in this view) on the medial surface of the fetlock, severe septic cellulitis, tenosynovitis, and arthritis leading to massive joint swelling.

The fetlock joint of the Friesian cow in 7.128 (with flexor tendons reflected) contains inspissated pus (*Arcanobacterium pyogenes*), but has minimal damage to the articular cartilage. In such cases joint infection often results from ascending digital sepsis. *Erysipelas* is also commonly isolated.

The longitudinal section of the metacarpus of a 7-week-old Angus heifer (7.129) shows skin necrosis, and infection has led to sepsis of the metacarpophalangeal (fetlock) joint. The skin necrosis had developed from overlong application of splints and a plaster cast (4 weeks) for the immobilization of a midshaft metacarpal fracture (A), which is seen to have healed.

In a case of septic arthritis of the elbow in the 14-month-old Holstein heifer in 7.130, brownish pus adheres to the joint surfaces. The articular surfaces, especially of the distal humerus, are severely eroded (A). Periarticular fibrosis is present.

Some cases of infection of major joints occur in adult cows and develop insidiously. This old cow from the Czech Republic with chronic infectious gonitis (7.131) had lost a lot of weight and was in obvious pain. Long-standing degenerative and proliferative changes had caused considerable enlargement of the stifle joint. *Brucella abortus* was recovered from the synovial fluid.

7.127. Severe septic swelling of left fore fetlock in calf (4 months old)

7.129. Secondary sepsis of fetlock joint spreading from skin necrosis (excessive splint pressure)

7.130. Septic arthritis of elbow in heifer (Holstein, 14 months old) (USA)

7.132. Bilateral tarsal bursitis and cellulitis

Such cows with an infectious, albeit nonseptic, arthritis should be culled.

Conditions of the hock region

Hock trauma is commonly seen in confinement housing systems with inadequate bedding, and especially when the cubicle/free-stall size and design are deficient. Solid, horizontal, wooden dividing rails and vertical uprights often cause injuries, although lack of bedding and a slippery surface, leading to abrasive trauma as the weight-bearing limb moves over the floor surface during rising and sitting, are the major causes. Trauma may also develop secondary to digital lameness, when cows are recumbent for long periods or have difficulty in rising. Many forms of hock swelling and injury nevertheless cause little or no lameness.

Tarsal bursitis and cellulitis

Clinical features: lateral swellings over the subcutaneous bursae of both hocks (also called cellulitis) are common in cattle housed on concrete (7.132). Carpal hygroma (7.147) causes a similar foreleg problem. The hair loss results from chronic abrasion. A horizontal section through an affected hock (7.133) shows a discrete discolored cavity (A) lined with granulation tissue. The synovia-like fluid is sterile. The majority of cases are not infected. An outward deviation of the digits (cow-hocked) often contributes to the development of tarsal bursitis.

Cellulitis develops when the skin barrier is broken and the wound becomes infected and discharges pus (7.134). The swelling then tends to be more diffuse than in aseptic bursitis, the joint capsule may become involved, and marked pain and lameness result. In another cow the right hock and adjacent limb are very swollen with an extensive cellulitis (7.135). The injury resulted from a puncture wound which introduced infection into the subcutaneous tissues. Although such animals do become very lame, this cow recovered after antibiotic therapy.

7

7.131. Chronic infectious gonitis in thin Friesian cow (Czech Republic)

7.133. Cavity (A) with fluid and granulation tissue in tarsal bursitis (cross-section)

7.134. Tarsal cellulitis with discharging track

Differential diagnosis: infectious (septic) tarsitis, tarsal fracture.

Management: unless very large, noninfected lesions are best treated conservatively by simply removing the animal from the traumatic environment and allowing natural resolution, which commonly occurs when cows

7.136. Medial tarsal hygroma, bilateral

go out to pasture at the end of the winter. If winter-housed, cows should be put onto straw bedding for several weeks. Larger lesions can be drained by sterile aspiration, although the puncture wound produced can lead to secondary infection. If a sterile bursitis is lanced, secondary infection is a common sequel. Cellulitis lesions require prolonged and aggressive antibiotic therapy.

Medial tarsal hygroma

Clinical features: the bilateral synovial swelling in 7.136 is fluctuating, painless, and its size results in slight mechanical lameness. The condition is sporadic and may result from trauma on the edge of the cubicle curb.

A traumatic abrasive sore is seen on the medial surface of the hock (7.137) in milking dairy cows. Again the edge of the freestall curb may be the initiating factor. Freestall discomfort with the cow lying with her leg extended back into the passage may be a trigger factor.

7.135. Severe tarsal cellulitis with gross proximal swelling

7.137. Medial hock sore

7.138. Tenosynovitis of tarsal sheath ("capped hock") in cow (Holstein, 3 years old)

Tenosynovitis of the tarsal sheath ("capped hock")

Clinical features: a firm swelling surrounds the point of the hock of this 3-year-old Holstein cow (7.138) and extends distally toward the tibiotarsal joint. Six months previously, the cow had fallen through a metal floor grid, sustaining an open wound involving the medial aspect of the tarsal sheath. Sepsis resulted, but the wound eventually healed with fibrosis.

Gastrocnemius trauma

Clinical features: trauma to the gastrocnemius muscle–tendon group arises sporadically from struggling, as when a cow with hypocalcemia (milk fever) attempts to stand following a period of recumbency. Rare cases are associated with vitamin D deficiency and aphosphorosis. The prognosis is generally hopeless, except in young animals, where external support may permit slow healing by fibrosis. Two manifestations of gastrocnemius rupture are shown. The first (7.139) shows a dropped hock and swelling of the gastrocnemius muscle belly in a Shorthorn heifer.

The Friesian cow in 7.140 has a complete bilateral rupture, cannot stand, and bears weight on the plantar surfaces of the hock. The appearance is similar to avulsion of the epiphyses of the os calcis, whereby the gastrocnemius muscle–tendon is intact. Another form of gastrocnemius injury is traumatic transection, as shown in the 2-year-old Friesian heifer in 7.141. This injury arises from a slicing action and can be very severe. The wound is invariably infected. Since both gastrocnemius and superficial flexor tendons are involved, weightbearing is made impossible.

Differential diagnosis: fracture of the os calcis, rupture of the gastrocnemius muscle belly.

Management: most cases of complete rupture or gastrocnemius transection fail to heal as a result of

7.139. Dropped hock and gastrocnemius rupture in heifer (Shorthorn)

continuing attempts at weightbearing. In smaller growing stock splintage in noninfected cases may permit recovery in some weeks.

Peripheral paralyses

One form of peripheral paralysis (obturator) has already been illustrated (7.91–7.92). Other types of nerve damage are illustrated in the following section.

Sciatic paralysis (L_6, S_{1-2} nerve roots)

Left sciatic paralysis resulted from the accidental (iatrogenic) perineural injection of an antibiotic solution into the deep gluteal region of this Angus heifer (7.142). Long-acting antibiotic preparations are commonly implicated.

7.140. Bilateral complete gastrocnemius rupture (Friesian)

7.143. Right femoral paralysis in calf (Simmental, 4 days old)

7.141. Traumatic transection of gastrocnemius tendon in heifer (Friesian, 2 years old)

Sciatic paralysis occasionally develops following prolonged recumbency resulting from parturient paresis. Severe ischemic muscle necrosis is evident around the damaged nerve (see downer cow, p. 121).

Femoral paralysis (L$_{4-6}$ nerve roots)

The flexed stifle cannot be extended to allow weightbearing, owing to dysfunction of the quadriceps group in this 4-day-old Simmental calf (7.143). Skin sensation was absent over part of the medial aspect of the thigh. A secondary lateral patellar luxation is sometimes present (7.114). A hollowed-out appearance of the quadriceps muscle (atrophy) is seen after about 7–10 days. Neonatal cases are the most common and their pathogenesis is often unclear. Fetal hyperextension caused by excessive traction during delivery, muscular compression, and ischemic anoxia may account for the clinical signs.

Differential diagnosis: lateral patellar luxation.

Peroneal paralysis (cranial division of sciatic nerve roots)

Peroneal paralysis is a common postpartum injury, as in the 6-year-old Friesian in 7.144. The stance resulted from paralysis of the hock flexors and digital extensors. Paresis or paralysis may persist for days or weeks, or occasionally indefinitely. The peroneal nerve is most susceptible to damage over the lateral surface of the stifle joint, and injury with subsequent paralysis is therefore seen following recumbency on a hard surface. Most are unilateral. Knuckling may be so pronounced as to cause abrasion of the dorsal aspect of the fetlock leading to joint damage.

Differential diagnosis: tibial paralysis (not shown), sciatic paralysis or paresis.

Management: avoid hard and slippery surfaces which could result in further injury.

7.142. Sciatic paralysis from inadvertent iatrogenic injection

7.144. Bilateral peroneal paralysis in cow (Friesian, 6 years old)

7.145. Radial paralysis in cow (Holstein)

Radial paralysis (C$_{7-8}$, T$_1$ nerve roots)

This mature Holstein cow (7.145) shows a dropped elbow, flexed carpus and fetlock, and an inability to bear weight. The cow had been maintained under general anesthesia, in right lateral recumbency on a padded table for 2 hours. Paralysis was immediately evident on standing but the gait was normal 2 days later.

Differential diagnosis: humeral fracture.

Brachial plexus injury (C$_6$–T$_1$ nerve roots)

The elbow of the Friesian cow in 7.146 was dropped, but the forelimb could be advanced for some limited weight-bearing. This injury can result from severe abduction of the forelimb, e.g., when falling after mounting a cow in estrus. Some radial paralysis (the radial nerve being one component of the plexus) was present.

Management: if weather conditions permit, keep the cow at pasture to promote exercise and avoid further injuries, otherwise place into bedded loose box. Avoid self-trauma from struggling to rise (sciatic), or abrasion to dorsal aspect of fetlock (radial). NSAIDs reduce discomfort.

7.146. Brachial plexus damage with dropped elbow in cow (Friesian)

7.147. Massive bilateral carpal hygromata (Czech Republic)

Miscellaneous locomotor conditions

Carpal hygroma

Definition: large fluid-filled sac on the front of the carpus.

Clinical features: carpal hygromata rarely reach the size seen in the forelegs of this old Friesian cow (7.147). They are usually bilateral, contain thin, serum-like material, and cause little or no lameness. Like tarsal bursitis (7.132), carpal hygromata result from repeated contusions on hard surfaces (concrete) in poorly designed housing, or, rarely today, from brucellosis.

Management: transfer to straw yard or pasture for slow resolution.

Spastic paresis ("Elso heel")

Definition: uncommon progressive hind limb extensor spasms of unknown etiology.

Clinical features: in this 6-month-old Friesian heifer (7.148) the left hock is overextended, and the gastrocnemius tendon and muscle were tense on palpation. This inherited condition, sporadically seen in both dairy and beef breeds, affects one or both hind limbs, producing a progressive disability that starts at 2–9 months old. Surgical correction can be performed, but is not recommended in breeding animals.

Differential diagnosis: dorsal patellar luxation, joint ill, gonitis, localized spinal trauma or space-occupying lesion.

Management: surgery to permit animal to be fattened, otherwise early culling.

7

7.148. Spastic paresis ("Elso heel") in heifer (Friesian, 6 months old)

Hip dysplasia

Definition: a progressive and probably inherited, bilateral, degenerative joint disease, seen in several beef breeds including the Aberdeen Angus and the Hereford.

Clinical features: the yearling Hereford bull in 7.149 has severe atrophy of the hindquarters. The forefeet are placed caudally and the hindfeet cranially to increase the proportion of weight borne by the forequarters. The acetabulum of another Hereford bull (7.150) shows the extensive cartilaginous erosion and areas of bone loss that result from this degenerative process. The clinical signs start at 2–18 months old. Hip dysplasia is generally progressive.

Differential diagnosis: osteochondrosis dissecans of stifle.

Osteochondrosis dissecans (OCD)

OCD occasionally causes a degenerative and aseptic joint problem of unknown etiology in groups of young,

7.150. Hip dysplasia: erosion and bone loss in acetabulum

fast-growing beef cattle. The opened joints of a yearling Angus crossbred steer (7.151) that had chronic, bilaterally enlarged shoulder joints, leading to lameness and poor growth, show loss of cartilage and subchondral bone (A), and periarticular fibrosis (B). Joints commonly involved are stifles, hocks, and shoulder.

Differential diagnosis: septic polyarthritis, hip dysplasia, muscle dystrophy.

Management: the development of OCD is poorly understood, but it has been associated with rapid growth rates on high-concentrate diets in the young animal, insufficient exercise, inadequate mineralization of the diet, and suboptimal floor surfaces. Several such factors need thorough investigation for management advice on prevention.

Septic myositis (popliteal abscess)

Clinical features: the massive swelling seen in the right thigh of this 2-year-old Simmental bull (7.152) caused a moderate lameness. The lighter area had been clipped for exploratory puncture. The swelling contained

7.149. Hip dysplasia in yearling bull, showing severe wasting (Hereford)

7.151. Osteochondrosis dissecans (OCD) of shoulder joint in steer (Angus cross 1 year old) (USA)

7.152. Massive septic myositis (popliteal abscess) in bull (Simmental, 2 years old)

12 liters of pus (isolate: *Arcanobacterium pyogenes*). For a further discussion, see popliteal abscess (3.67).

Management: ensure adequate drainage following a long incision, and initially irrigation and gentle curettage of the focus.

Rupture of the ventral serrate muscle

The right scapula of the mature Flemish Maas-Rijn-Ijssel cow in 7.153 projects above the thoracic spine owing to the rupture of the ventral serrate and subscapularis muscles. The scapula returns to its normal anatomical position when the leg is not bearing weight. In mature cattle the etiology is probably chronic muscle degeneration and atrophy.

Management: although it is a cosmetic blemish, affected cows can easily be retained to the end of a lactation.

7.153. Right ventral serrate muscle rupture in cow (FMR) (Belgium)

7.154. White muscle disease ("flying scapula") in two beef steers

White muscle disease (enzootic muscle dystrophy, "flying scapula")

Definition: muscle degeneration caused by vitamin E and/or selenium deficiency in which an accumulation of free peroxide radicals leads to muscle degeneration and a calcium deposition necrosis.

Clinical features: clinical signs are often seen following spring turn-out when a sudden increase in exercise and general muscle stress is combined with a dramatic intake of FFA in lush springtime grazing. This is particularly the case if poor winter feeding had induced a vitamin E/selenium deficiency. Affected cattle may show lameness, general locomotor impairment, dyspnea if the diaphragm is affected, and sudden death from cardiac degeneration. In 7.154 ventral serrate and subscapular muscle function has been lost allowing the scapula to rise above the thoracic spine in the two beef steers. Note the wide-based foreleg stance to accommodate the abnormal support mechanism. The heart of a calf with white muscle disease (7.155) has extensive pale grayish areas (A) on the epicardium, typically extending into the myocardium. There may also be endothelial plaques. The cardiac shape is globular following chronic hypertrophy (7.155). White muscle lesions, usually bilateral, are also seen at autopsy in skeletal muscle and diaphragm.

7.155. White muscle disease: globular heart with greyish patches (A)

7.156. Foreign body (wire) encircling metatarsus in bull (Limousin, 2 years old)

Management: provision of a balanced diet and where necessary supplementation with vitamin E and/or selenium. Requirements increase with rapid growth rates and high-oil diets, especially high polyunsaturated fatty acids (PUFAs). Individual affected animals respond well to parenteral therapy with vitamin E and selenium.

Foreign body around the metatarsus

In 7.156 a piece of wire is being removed from a characteristic, deep, circumferential, granulating wound of the metatarsal soft tissues. The 2-year-old Limousin bull was moderately lame and recovered rapidly.

Differential diagnosis: other forms of wounds.

Management: adequate restraint and deep exploration with forceps down to metatarsus to detect and remove metal wire.

Distal limb gangrene: traumatic origin

In 7.157 a clear line demarcates the dead from the healthy skin. The Holstein cow had caught her leg at the metacarpal level in a stanchion chain, and was found recumbent the following morning, with the chain still in place. A few days later the skin was dry and painless. It sloughed 3 weeks later, together with the distal soft tissues and hoof horn capsule, necessitating euthanasia. Compare skin changes in 7.156.

Management: early culling.

Fescue foot gangrene

Definition: fescue foot is caused by an ergot-like toxin, consumed by cattle grazing certain endophyte-infested strains of tall fescue grasses in many states of the USA, as well as in New Zealand, Italy, Australia, and Orkney (UK).

Clinical features: in the 11-month-old Hereford steer in 7.158, the dark areas of skin on the hind pasterns are

7.157. Distal limb gangrene following stanchion chain injury (USA)

dry gangrene. A sharply defined oblique line (A) extending over the fetlock separates the dead from the normal skin. Skin has also separated from the coronary band to expose infected subcutis (B). The upper (right) limb shows a pink area where the gangrenous skin has sloughed. The ear tips and tail may also become gangrenous. The problem affects several younger cattle in a group, all of which are at risk.

Differential diagnosis: ergotism (7.159), frostbite (3.73), trauma (7.157), salmonellosis (2.26).

7.158. Fescue foot gangrene in steer (Hereford, 11 months old) (USA)

Management: change of pasture if practical, or confinement and feeding of endophyte-free hay. The individual case cannot be cured.

Ergot gangrene

Definition: ergotism results from ingestion of the parasitic fungus *Claviceps purpurea* on hay, grain, or seeded pastures.

Clinical features: gangrene of the extremities resulting from the ingestion of ergot-infested cereals and other feeds is a worldwide problem. The clinical features resemble fescue foot (7.158). The lower limb and tail tip are affected in the yearling heifer in 7.159. Gangrenous skin is sloughing from the left metatarsal region, and a similar line of demarcation is seen in the right leg. The distal 25 cm of the tail is twisted, moist and gangrenous. More advanced changes in the feet are shown in 7.160. The left foot has almost sloughed at the pastern, and the distal third of the tail is detached.

Differential diagnosis: fescue foot (7.158), frostbite (3.73), trauma (7.157), salmonellosis (2.26).

Hyena disease

Definition: a rare chondrodystrophy of the hindlimb bones and lumbar vertebrae of unknown etiology, often accompanied by aggressive behavior.

Clinical features: this severely affected, 3-year-old French Friesian cow (7.161) has a hyena-like silhouette, with underdevelopment of the hindquarters. Calves are normal at birth, and manifest the initial signs of the disease at 6–10 months. Compared with a normal tibia of a 2-year-old animal (7.162, left), the tibia of an

7.160. Severe digital and tail gangrene due to ergot

7.161. Hyena disease in cow (Friesian, 3 years old) (France)

7

7.159. Ergot gangrene in metatarsal area of both legs (USA)

7.162. Hyena disease: normal (left) and shortened tibia at autopsy (France)

affected individual (22 months) is considerably short-ened, although the width and articular surface area are comparable. The condition is thought to result from a bone dysplasia.

Management: incurable.

Deficiency diseases

Rickets

Definition: caused by a calcium, phosphorus, or vitamin D deficiency, rickets involves a failure of calcifica-tion of osteoid and cartilage in young growing animals.

7.164. Phosphorus deficiency ("osteomalacia", "peg-leg") in stunted emaciated steer (Brazil)

Clinical features: swelling and pain generally involve all the major limb joints. In the 6-month-old Holstein heifer in 7.163 the fetlock is enlarged due to widening of the distal metatarsal physis. The articular surfaces are normal. The calf is lame. Poorly mineralized high-concentrate diets that promote rumen acidosis can lead to a type of rickets producing spontaneous fractures in rapidly growing cattle.

Differential diagnosis: copper deficiency (7.171), epiphysitis. See also spinal compression fracture (7.94).

Management: dietary correction.

Phosphorus deficiency (osteomalacia, "peg-leg")

Definition: impaired mineralization of bones of adult cattle, with excess osteoid accumulation, caused by phosphorus and/or vitamin D deficiency. Phosphorus deficiency is the most common mineral deficiency worldwide.

Clinical features: affected cattle are unthrifty, have a poor appetite, and walk stiffly. The Brazilian steer in 7.164 is stunted, extremely emaciated, and walked with

7.165. Phosphorus deficiency or osteomalacia in cow (Zebu (Gir)) (Brazil)

great difficulty. The local term for this severe aphospho-rosis is "entreva." The Brazilian Zebu (Gir) cow (7.165) is eating a bone, demonstrating pica; other bones litter the ground. This habit may result in botulism (12.69). A carcass of a phosphorus-deficient animal from the Aus-tralian outback has multiple fractured ribs that are so soft they can easily be cut with a knife (7.166). A phosphorus

7.163. Rickets: enlarged fetlocks in lame heifer (Holstein, 6 months old) (Canada)

7.166. Multiple fractured ribs indicative of phosphorus deficiency (Australia)

7.167. Copper deficiency ("pine") in heifer with brownish coat (Hereford cross)

7.169. Copper deficiency with spectacled appearance in calf (Holstein cross)

deficiency in young cattle causes rickets (7.163) with slow growth and joint deformities.

Differential diagnosis: other mineral deficiencies, e.g., calcium, copper, and cobalt, and starvation.

Management: the easiest and cheapest prophylaxis is the supply of a phosphatic mineral supplement in troughs or boxes protected from the rain. In Australian beef cattle, due to low soil phosphorus levels, a phosphorus concentrate may be needed all the time. Problem of supply of supplements is common in range conditions.

Copper deficiency (hypocuprosis, "pine")

Definition: abnormally low blood and tissue copper levels.

Clinical features: the crossbred Hereford heifer in 7.167 is unthrifty and has enlarged fetlocks and a characteristic brownish tinge to the hair coat. (The Hereford also has lice.) The loss of hair and hair pigment (7.168) may produce a "spectacled" appearance, as seen in the crossbred Holstein/Friesian calf in 7.169, which also shows coarse hair typical of copper deficiency. Bone

7.170. Copper deficiency with poor growth and hair (Brazil)

fragility and anemia are other clinical features. The Brazilian cows in 7.170 show poor growth, poor hair coat, and loss of pigment. The fetlock joint enlargement (7.171) is due to widening and irregularity of the distal metacarpal physes, as seen in the radiographs (7.172) of an affected animal (left) compared with a normal animal (right). Similar radiographic changes are seen in the digits. Other cattle may become stunted, developing bowed legs, contracted tendons, and kyphosis. Excluding phosphorus deficiency, a deficiency of copper may be the most severe

7.168. Copper deficiency

7.171. Copper deficiency: widened metacarpal physes causing enlarged fetlock joint

7.172. Copper deficiency: radiograph of fetlock (left affected, right normal)

7.173. Manganese deficiency with joint deformities in neonate (Hereford) (Canada)

mineral limitation to grazing livestock in extensive tropical regions.

Differential diagnosis: aphosphorosis (7.164), rickets (7.163), cobalt deficiency (7.174).

Management: copper supplements.

Manganese deficiency

Definition: abnormally low blood manganese levels in dam or offspring leading to various skeletal deformities and infertility.

Clinical features: this Hereford neonate (7.173) cannot stand owing to a congenital twisting and flexion of the enlarged fetlock joints. Various other skeletal abnormalities are also present. These changes resulted from a severe manganese deficiency in the dam during gestation. In a 100-head Hereford herd in Canada, of the 5–10% of calves that were born with abnormalities, this calf was among the most severely affected. Following external splintage, many calves recovered from tendon contracture.

Management: supplementary manganese to pregnant beef cattle at risk, limb splintage where needed in young calves, and good nursing.

Cobalt deficiency ("pine", enzootic marasmus)

Definition: inadequate intake of cobalt over prolonged period, causing poor weight gain and anorexia.

Clinical features: the Brazilian Zebu cattle are depressed, emaciated, eat little, and have a poor hair coat (7.174). They are also anemic. Visual evidence of cobalt deficiency is nonspecific, resembling the signs of semistarvation. Young animals are more susceptible. Diagnosis may ultimately rest on the response to cobalt supplementation.

Differential diagnosis: aphosphorosis (osteomalacia) (7.164), hypocuprosis (7.167), parasitism, low feed intake.

Management: confirmation of deficiency by biochemical analysis of blood and other tissues, also feed, followed by adequate access to mineral supplements.

7.174. Cobalt deficiency ("pine"): emaciated poor hair coat (Zebu) (Brazil)

Ocular disorders

Introduction

Disorders of the eye are relatively easily seen and photographed. The disorders may be congenital, nutritional, infectious, traumatic, or neoplastic in origin. Examples of each are illustrated. Some conditions, e.g., infectious bovine keratoconjunctivitis (IBK), occur worldwide, and may be a significant cause of economic loss. Pain associated with the active phase of disease restricts feeding and leads to weight loss. If sight is lost, affected animals are less able to forage, particularly under extensive ranch conditions, and they are more susceptible to predators.

Congenital disorders

Although by definition congenital abnormalities are present at birth, some may not be recognized until the calf is much older. Strabismus (squint) is a typical example. Congenital disorders may be genetic, and therefore inherited, or they may be caused by environmental factors. Some abnormalities have more than one cause. For example, congenital cataract may be inherited, or it may have been caused by maternal BVD infection during pregnancy. The cause of many abnormalities is unknown. Congenital disorders in organs other than the eye are described in Chapter 1.

BVD/MD, discussed under "Alimentary disorders" (p. 54) can give rise to congenital or acquired ocular changes. Congenital BVD/MD can cause teratogen-induced retinal necrosis and degeneration, focal capsular cataract, as well as optic nerve gliosis, microphthalmos (see below) and optic neuritis. 8.1 shows retinal changes in a calf associated with the teratogenic effects of BVD/MD virus. There is marked attenuation of many retinal blood vessels, retinal hyper-reflectivity and a patchy yellow pigmentary disturbance.

Anophthalmos (anophthalmia); microphthalmos (microphthalmia)

Definition: anophthalmos is a developmental absence of the eye; microphthalmos is an abnormal smallness of one or both eyes.

Clinical features: the two examples illustrate both abnormalities. The left eye of the Guernsey heifer in 8.2 has a small orbit and there is no evidence of the globe. Note that the entire orbit appears collapsed and smaller, compared with the normal right eye. This condition can be inherited. A Jersey cow with microphthalmos (8.3) and prolapse of orbital fat had possibly had an insult to the eye in calfhood, leading to this shrunken globe (*phthisis bulbi*).

Cataract

Definition: opacity of the lens or its capsule, or both, present at birth or acquired from trauma or systemic disease.

8.1. Retinal dysplasia in BVD

8.4. Cataract, bilateral, (Hereford cross, 4 days old)

8.2. Anophthalmos in left eye of heifer (Guernsey)

8

Clinical features: both eyes of the 4-day-old Hereford crossbred calf in 8.4 were affected and the animal was totally blind. In other animals, only one eye may be affected, or the cataract may not cause total loss of vision. Congenital cataract is not normally progressive. Cattle cope with blindness remarkably well and can be reared in confinement systems. They quickly learn to remain within the group, although handling can be difficult. Blind dairy cows will learn to follow the herd to and from pasture. Congenital cataract may be inherited, or

8.5. Congenital nuclear cataract in calf resulting from maternal BVD infection (Friesian)

may result from the teratogenic effects of maternal BVD infection during early/mid pregnancy. 8.5 shows a congenital nuclear cataract in a young Friesian calf.

Note in acquired cataract the two large synechiae (adhesions of the iris to the cornea), and the opacity and wrinkling of the lens in the Guernsey cow in 8.6.

8.3. Microphthalmos in cow (Jersey)

8.6. Acquired cataract in cow (Guernsey)

8.7. Coloboma involving retina in cow

Cataracts may be secondary to inflammatory processes within the eye, when they can be progressive. In contrast, congenital cataracts (8.4) are rarely progressive.

Coloboma

Definition: a coloboma is a congenital cleft caused by failure of the embryonic optic fissure to close.

Clinical features: it can occur in the eyelids, iris, lens, or, as shown in 8.7, the retina. Note the pale area devoid of functional retinal cells. The condition is inherited in certain breeds of cattle (e.g., Charolais), but vision is not normally impaired.

Dermoid

Definition: an uncommon tumor of developmental origin containing various tissues such as hair follicles, various glandular structures, and nerve elements, located often on the cornea, conjunctiva, and eyelids.

Clinical features: a typical dermoid is seen in a 4-month-old Friesian heifer (8.8). The tumor is attached to the conjunctiva of the lower lid and presents long hairs, which led to the presenting sign of unilateral epiphora.

Management: most ocular dermoids can be resected surgically. Recurrence is unlikely.

Strabismus ("squint")

Definition: involuntary deviation of the eye.

Clinical features: strabismus may be convergent (esotopia), when the visual axes of the eyes converge more than is required for normal vision, or divergent. It may involve one or both eyes. The globe is deviated from its

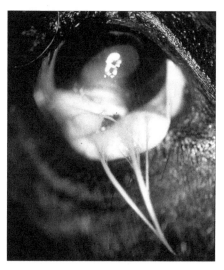

8.8. Dermoid attached to conjunctiva in heifer (Friesian, 4 months old)

proper axis due to excessive tension in opposing extraocular muscles. 8.9 shows convergent strabismus in the left eye of a Hereford cross heifer. Exophthalmos with strabismus may be inherited, although it is often unnoticed until 6–9 months old, and it is frequently progressive. Some animals may become so badly affected that total impairment of vision results.

Neonatal corneal opacity

A reduction in intraocular pressure in stillborn calves leads to cloudiness in the cornea and indicates that the calf has died at least 12 hours before birth. In the stillborn Charolais calf in 8.10 the eyeball is also slightly sunken in the socket.

8

8.9. Convergent strabismus ("squint") in heifer (Hereford cross)

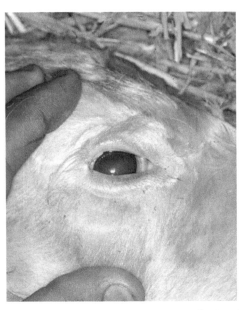

8.10.   Neonatal corneal opacity in stillborn calf (Charolais)

Acquired disorders

Vitamin A deficiency

In young growing animals, vitamin A deficiency blindness is associated with stenosis of the optic foramen and consequent pressure on the optic nerve. The pupil becomes dilated and degenerative changes may be seen on the retina (8.11). For comparison, 8.12 shows a normal fundus. The optic disc is pale and enlarged, with indistinct margins (papilledema). White mottling of the nontapetal area suggests chorioretinal degeneration.

8.11.   Vitamin A deficiency: degenerative changes in retina (blind steer) (Canada)

8.12.   Normal fundus

The steer was blind. The diet had been barley straw, rolled barley and, occasionally, poor-quality hay.

Management: ensure diets of cereals, straw, and similar feeds are adequately supplemented with vitamin A, especially for rapidly growing stock.

Conjunctivitis

Mild conjunctivitis is seen clinically as epiphora. Typically, a wet, black-stained facial area radiates from the medial canthus. More advanced cases (8.13) show a degree of photophobia. Purulent conjunctivitis (8.14) may also be seen. Caused by a variety of infections and irritants, conjunctivitis and epiphora commonly occur in association with other diseases, e.g., calf pneumonia, IBR (5.2), IBK (8.15), and ocular foreign body (8.27).

Infectious bovine keratoconjunctivitis (IBK, infectious ophthalmia, "New Forest disease" or "pinkeye")

Definition and pathogenesis: a bacterial infection caused by *Moraxella bovis*, IBK produces blepharospasm, conjunctivitis, keratitis, and corneal ulceration.

8.13.   Conjunctivitis and photophobia

8.14. Purulent conjunctivitis

8.16. IBK with corneal opacity and pannus

Clinical features: in mild cases, corneal ulceration may not be apparent and the only clinical signs are epiphora and partial blepharospasm. Typically the ulcer is in the center of the cornea and may be superficial or erode deeply into the stroma as shown in a more advanced case (8.15). Conjunctivitis is always present. The condition is very painful, leading to photophobia, blepharospasm, and epiphora. Early (adventitious) corneal vascularization has developed into pannus formation in 8.15. Later stages (8.16) develop corneal opacity due to increased intraocular pressure, and a bright red circumferential rim of pannus (A) progressing from the corneoscleral junction to fill the central ulcer. The pannus will regress when healing is complete.

Pannus formation does not occur with shallow, superficial lesions, where the ulcer is seen in a localized area of corneal opacity (8.17). If corneal rupture does not occur, healing may be complete, or may leave a small corneal scar (A), as seen towards the medial canthus in 8.18. Partial sight has been regained. The circular plaque (B) on the cornea is an artifact caused by flash photography.

8.17. IBK with central ulcer

8.15. Infectious bovine keratoconjunctivitis (IBK) with severe corneal ulcer

8.18. IBK with scar (A)

8.19.   IBK with perforating ulcer and staphyloma

Deep ulcers may perforate through to the aqueous humor. In 8.19, tissue from the iris plugs the ruptured ulcer and can be seen as a red ring protruding from the surface of the cornea. This is a staphyloma. More advanced cases lose their red appearance and some may eventually heal, but they leave an opaque, scarred cornea (8.20). At this stage most cases are nonpainful and do not trouble the animal, although there may be glaucoma from impaired drainage of the aqueous humor.

Differential diagnosis: diagnosis is easily made on ocular signs especially if several cattle are affected. Differentials include bovine iritis (8.35–8.37), malignant catarrhal fever, bluetongue, and foreign bodies (usually peripheral, see 8.27), parasites (8.29), and IBR. *Moraxella bovis* infection can be confirmed on culture in doubtful cases. Note that IBK and IBR eye lesions can rarely be present in the same animal.

Management: bright sunlight, dry, dusty, and irritant conditions, flies, and a tight stocking density are all predisposing factors. Separation of affected animals is advisable, preferably in the shade. *M. bovis* is susceptible to

8.21.   Hypopyon (pus in anterior chamber) in calf (4 weeks old)

various antibiotics which may be administered subconjunctivally, topically, or parenterally. Surgery (third eyelid flap) may help severely affected individuals. The efficacy of *M. bovis* bacterins is still disputed.

Hypopyon

Definition: pus in the anterior chamber.

Clinical features: this 4-week-old calf (8.21) was dull, pyrexic, and anorexic due to calfhood septicemia resulting from colostrum deficiency. Note the white blood cells in the anterior chamber. This calf recovered following antibiotics and NSAIDs. *Histophilus somni* septicemia can produce blindness from retinal hemorrhages and edema (8.22).

Ocular trauma

Clinical features: although the eye is well protected within the bony orbit and by the rapid reflex closure of the lids to approaching foreign bodies, traumatic eye lesions are common, particularly those due to incoming

8.20.   IBK with residual scarred cornea and glaucoma

8.22.   Hypopyon, retinal hemorrhages, and edema (*Histophilus somni* infection) (Canada)

8.23. Ocular trauma with scleral congestion, indistinct pupil, and medial corneal opacity in cow (Guernsey)

8.24. Scleral hemorrhage in 4 day-old Holstein calf

objects. Irritation due to dust or ultraviolet light may produce keratitis and conjunctivitis. The Guernsey cow in 8.23 has a congested scleral conjunctiva (seen below the upper eyelid), an indistinct pupil, and mild corneal opacity at the medial canthus, probably the result of a blow. The calf in 8.24 has marked scleral hemorrhage following dystocia. In a downer cow, resulting from severe dystocia, 8.25 shows perforation of cornea, and prolapse of the lens and iris. Another cow (8.26) shows

8.26. Conjunctival edema

the secondary results of external trauma to the head: opaque corneal striations, early hyphema, and severe conjunctival edema.

Management: most cases resolve completely within a few days. If persistent, a further check for a foreign body should be made before starting topical therapy.

Ocular foreign body

Clinical features: grass seeds or other plant material may become lodged in the conjunctiva and, as the eyeball moves, repeatedly traumatize the area to produce erosion and ulceration. Cattle reaching up to feed from overhead hay racks are particularly at risk. In 8.27 a small fragment of plant material (A) is embedded in the corneal surface near the lateral canthus. Note the surrounding early peripheral keratitis and corneal opacity. Keratitis with early corneal ulceration is seen in the more advanced case in 8.28. Most of the foreign body is lodged in the lateral canthus, with one small fragment protruding across the cornea.

Management: following good restraint and possibly use of a topical local anesthetic, the foreign body can be removed manually or with fine, blunt-tipped forceps. Topical therapy should be given for several days. Small

8.25. Perforation of cornea, and prolapse of lens and iris

8.27. Ocular foreign body: embedded plant material (A)

8.28. Ocular foreign body with keratitis and early corneal ulceration

8.30. Prolapsed eyeball (proptosis) in cow (Ayrshire)

foreign bodies that become embedded in the cornea and produce a keratitis will often resolve spontaneously over time.

Thelazia ("eyeworm")

Definition: spiruroid worm (e.g., *T. rhodesii*) of family *Thelaziidae* which parasitizes the lacrimal duct and conjunctival sac of cattle, being deposited in the sac by flies as the intermediate host (*Musca* spp.).

Clinical features: infection causes chronic conjunctivitis, lacrimation, blepharospasm, and keratitis. 8.29 shows white *Thelazia* larvae floating in tear secretion in the lower conjunctival sac. Diagnosis is made on inspection.

8.29. Thelazia ("eyeworm") larvae in tear secretion

Differential diagnosis: IBK (8.15), bovine iritis (8.35), ocular trauma (8.27, 8.28).

Management: mechanical removal with forceps after instilling a local anesthetic solution. Prevention is by levamisole and ivermectin with doramectin, along with control measures against face flies.

Prolapse of the eyeball (proptosis)

Definition: forward displacement or bulging of the eye.

Clinical features: an infrequent condition caused by trauma to the head. In the Ayrshire cow in 8.30, note the congested and edematous sclera, and the eyeball protruding beyond the lids.

Management: under sedation and local anesthesia the eyeball can be returned to its socket. If held in place for 4–5 days by suturing the lids together, most cases (as in 8.30) resolve well.

Eyelid laceration

Clinical features: lacerations of the lower eyelids are fairly common. They are often caused by an animal rubbing the head and catching an eyelid on projections from troughs, buildings, or fragments of wire. In the Angus heifer in 8.31, the lower-lid injury near the lateral canthus was sustained several days previously and was healing well.

Management: sometimes the resultant rough eyelid edge leads to incomplete lid closure with persistent low-grade corneal ulceration and lacrimation. More severe cases should therefore benefit from suturing.

Entropion

Definition: inversion of the margin of an eyelid. A congenital or acquired condition.

8.31. Lacerated lower eyelid in heifer (Angus)

Clinical features: a Simmental bull, following uveitis (see bovine iritis, see p. 155) developed entropion of the right lower lid (8.32), where secondary corneal pannus formation is also evident. The entropion was of the spastic type and resolved following topical treatment.

Hyphema

Definition: hyphema is blood in the anterior chamber, with many possible causes such as trauma, clotting disorders, and sepsis.

Clinical features: in 8.33 note the fresh blood which has settled at the bottom of the anterior chamber. (See also bracken poisoning, 13.2.) A more advanced case is shown in 8.34, which illustrates corneal trauma resulting from a foreign body, with hyphema, conjunctivitis, and edema.

Management: many traumatic cases are bilateral and the animal has total but temporary loss of sight. Most cases resolve spontaneously over 2–3 weeks without treatment.

8.32. Entropion of lower lid and pannus in bull (Simmental)

8.33. Severe hyphema

Bovine iritis (uveitis, iridocyclitis, "silage eye")

Definition: inflammation of the anterior uveal tract (iris and ciliary body) is iridocyclitis, whilst posterior uveitis is inflammation of the ciliary body and choroid.

Clinical features: several neonatal (e.g., navel ill) as well as systemic diseases of growing and adult cattle may be associated with uveitis, such as malignant catarrhal fever, tuberculosis, and IBR. Bovine iritis has been more recently associated with *Listeria monocytogenes* infection and is possibly caused by the feeding of big-bale silage. One or both eyes are affected. Early cases (8.35) show an enlarged and wrinkled iris, leading to a central miotic pupil. Near the lateral canthus is a white endothelial plaque on the inner surface of the cornea (Descemet's membrane), with corneal opacity and early pannus formation. As the condition progresses (8.36), pannus develops circumferentially (A), with increasing corneal discoloration and opacity. In severe cases (8.37) the endothelial plaques produce a very irregular surface on the cornea and cause complete blindness.

Diagnosis: the association of close contact with big-bale silage and ocular disease in a group is characteristic.

8.34. Hyphema and conjunctival edema following skull concussion

8

8.35.   Early bovine iritis with enlarged wrinkled iris

8.36.   Bovine iritis with pannus (A) and opaque cornea

Other differentials include IBK (8.15–8.20) and ocular foreign body (8.27).

Management: even advanced cases (8.36, 8.37) recover following subconjunctival anti-inflammatory and antibiotic treatment. Major outbreaks occur when silage is cut at a fairly mature stage of grass growth. Feeding from round feeders and along wind-swept troughs, both of which increase eye contact with silage, increases disease risk.

8.37.   Severe bovine iritis with corneal plaque formation

Neoplastic conditions

Malignancy of the third eyelid (membrana nictitans) and the globe is common in cattle worldwide. Lymphosarcomas may occur within the globe itself or in the orbit, leading to prolapse of the globe. Papillomas have been occasionally reported.

Squamous cell carcinoma

Pathogenesis: squamous cell carcinoma (SCC) is the most common ocular neoplasm of cattle, and is seen particularly in mature white-headed beef cattle, such as the Hereford, and other breeds with little pigmentation around the eye (e.g., Simmental). The disease is associated with sunlight (ultraviolet light).

Clinical features: common sites for SCC include the lower lid, the third eyelid, and the corneoscleral junction of the globe. Often both eyes are affected to a varying degree. Small benign precursor lesions will often regress. The Hereford bull in 8.38 has SCC at several points along the eyelids (A), a grayish plaque, 10 mm in diameter, extending over the cornea from the corneoscleral junction (B), and early SCC in the third eyelid (C). In the Guernsey cow in 8.39 and the mature Friesian in 8.40, pink, neoplastic tissue protrudes from the third eyelid (membrana nictitans) at the medial canthus. In 8.40, other smaller lesions are evident on the lower lid and the corneal surface. There is a secondary superficial purulent infection. If neglected, about 10% of cases will eventually metastasize to the regional lymph nodes (resulting in slaughterhouse condemnation), and a small proportion to the lungs, as in 8.41. The multiple irregular pale areas are tumor tissue.

Differential diagnosis: IBK (8.15–8.20), periorbital lymphosarcoma (8.42).

Management: early third eyelid lesions are easily removed under sedation and local anesthesia using forceps and scissors. No suturing is required. More

8.38.   Squamous cell carcinoma (SCC) on eyelids, cornea, and third eyelid in bull (Hereford)

8.39. Neoplastic tissue (SCC) protruding from the third eyelid (membrana nictitans) at the medial canthus in cow (Guernsey)

8.40. Squamous cell carcinoma on third eyelid and lower lid (Friesian)

8.41. Lung metastases of squamous cell carcinoma

8.42. Lymphosarcoma as retroconjunctival mass (USA)

8

advanced cases require cryotherapy or total removal of the eyeball to avoid regional spread.

Lymphosarcoma (malignant lymphoma)

Definition: a malignant neoplasm of lymphatic tissue, lymphosarcoma can develop at several sites (abomasum, uterus). When in the eye, it usually presents as a retrobulbar mass with progressive expansion and spread.

Clinical features: in 8.42 a large neoplastic mass has produced a smooth, red, bulbous enlargement of the conjunctiva, compressing the eyeball towards the medial canthus (right). Ocular lymphosarcoma causes progressive exophthalmos.

Diagnosis: the tumor is almost invariably present in other sites, as clinical examination often reveals superficial, abdominal, and pelvic lymphadenopathy and other lymphosarcomatous foci. Biopsy and histopathology of the mass or enlarged lymph node can confirm diagnosis.

Management: affected cattle should be culled; secondary spread results in carcass condemnation.

Papilloma

In 8.43 a papilloma is attached to the third eyelid by a "stalk" and has a very irregular keratinized surface. It is much less common than an SCC, and is easy to remove surgically. Periocular papillomata ("warts") are frequently seen in groups of younger calves. 8.44 shows three mature papillomata originating from the skin of the eyelids at medial and lateral canthus. Several small papillomata can be seen distant from the eye. Other sites have been illustrated elsewhere (neck 3.45, penis 10.19, 10.20, teat 11.29–11.31). Periocular warts are purely a visual disfigurement and are best left alone to drop off eventually.

8.43.   Papilloma attached to third eyelid

8.44.   Periocular warts

8

Nervous disorders

Introduction

The diseases and disorders covered in this chapter have predominantly nervous signs. Consequently, a wide etiological range is covered including nutritional conditions (e.g., cerebrocortical necrosis), metabolic disorders (e.g., hypomagnesemia), bacterial and viral infections (e.g., listeriosis and rabies), parasites (e.g., *Coenurus cerebralis*), physical and traumatic incidents (lightning strike and electrocution), and miscellaneous conditions of uncertain etiology (e.g., bovine spongiform encephalopathy). However, other diseases with significant clinical nervous signs may be featured elsewhere and include tetanus (12.66–12.68), botulism (12.69), and lead poisoning (13.29).

Nervous conditions may be difficult to appreciate in "still" photographs, since their clinical assessment is based on changes in behavior, movement, gait, and stance. An understanding of the normal animal is therefore extremely important. Where problems of recognition occur, the text has been expanded in an attempt to describe those changes that cannot be photographed.

Cerebrocortical necrosis (polioencephalomalacia)

Etiology: cerebrocortical necrosis (CCN) is an induced thiamine deficiency caused by products of abnormal ruminal fermentation (thiaminases). Concentrate feeding leading to excessive growth of specific thiaminase 1 enzyme-secreting rumen bacteria is the most likely cause.

The syndrome can also be induced by feeding high levels of certain ammonium sulfate mixtures used as dietary urinary acidifiers for the prevention of urolithiasis (10.5–10.10).

Clinical features: CCN is seen most commonly in calves that are 2–6 months old, often following a dietary change when on high-concentrate rations. The Simmental crossbred calf in 9.1 has a characteristic "star-gazing" stance. Signs can be very variable depending on whether the onset is acute or subacute. Other signs include depression, ataxia, head-pressing (9.2), and cortical blindness. Autopsy lesions (9.3) are normally symmetrical and occur in the frontal, occipital, and parietal lobes. Congestion and yellow degeneration of the cortical gray matter (A) is seen, typically at the junction of the white and gray matter, particularly on the left and right extremities. Affected brains will fluoresce blue-green under ultraviolet light.

Differential diagnosis: acute lead poisoning, hypomagnesemia, brain abscess, vitamin A deficiency. Diagnosis is based on the clinical signs and response to thiamine therapy.

Management: multiple injections of thiamine hydrochloride, the first i.v., within a few hours of onset of signs, possibly also diuretics and/or dexamethasone, can lead to a marked improvement. Mortality in untreated animals can exceed 50%. Prevention involves avoidance of possible risk factors.

9.1. Cerebrocortical necrosis (CCN) "star-gazing" stance

9.2. CCN in Friesian calf showing head pressing

Metabolic diseases

Metabolic diseases are included in this chapter, since many of their presenting clinical signs are behavioral or nervous. Typically, such signs occur when homeostasis has been extended beyond physiological limits. Four conditions are illustrated: hypomagnesemia, hypocalcemia, acetonemia or ketosis, and fatty liver syndrome.

Hypomagnesemia ("grass staggers", "grass tetany")

Definition: hypomagnesemia is a complex metabolic disturbance involving lowered blood and cerebrospinal

9.3. Brain in CCN showing typical cortical changes (A) under UV light

9.4. Hypomagnesemia in collapsed cow with "staring" eye, dilated pupil, frothing, and sweaty coat (Friesian)

fluid (CSF) magnesium leading to hyperexcitability, muscle spasms, convulsions, and death, usually in adult lactating dairy or beef cows. In severe cases, death can occur within a few hours.

Clinical features: the Friesian cow in 9.4 fell and developed extensor spasm when being brought in for milking. Note the "staring" eye, dilated pupil, frothing at the mouth, and sweaty coat. In 9.5 the crossbred cow from Queensland, Australia, shows similar eye changes. The head and the hind legs are in extensor spasm. Violent paddling movements of the forelegs and head have resulted in loss of foliage, exposing the bare earth. Less severely affected cows may walk stiffly, are hypersensitive to touch and sound, and urinate often. Precipitated by stress and seen especially in temperate climates, the condition is induced by grazing magnesium-deficient or high-potassium pastures, and other pastures where magnesium uptake is poor. Concurrent hypocalcemia may be an exacerbating factor.

Differential diagnosis: hypocalcemia (9.6, 9.7), BSE (9.36–9.38) encephalitis, listeriosis (9.11, 9.12), ketosis (9.8).

Management: individual treatment involves sedation to control spasms and to prevent cardiac arrest, and subcutaneous injection of 25% solution of magnesium

9.5. Hypomagnesemia showing extensor spasm in cow (crossbred) (Australia)

9.6. Hypocalcemia showing recumbent cow with typical S-bend in neck (Friesian)

sulfate, possibly with calcium borogluconate. Small amounts of $MgSO_4$ can be given slowly i.v.

Prevention: maintain adequate intake of magnesium, either by sward management, buffer feeding, or by addition of magnesium salts to diet or drinking water.

Hypocalcemia ("milk fever", postparturient paresis)

Clinical features: hypocalcemia (9.6) occurs typically in older cows immediately pre- or postcalving. Early signs include hypersensitivity and increased excitability. Later, affected animals are unable to rise owing to lack of muscle power and poor nerve function. Note also the protruding anal sphincter (due to accumulation of feces in the rectum and increased intra-abdominal pressure), slight ruminal bloat (ruminal atony), and the typical "S-bend" in the neck (9.6). This is thought to be a self-righting response, as the animal attempts to avoid full lateral recumbency. Some affected cows lie with their head resting on their flank (9.7).

Differential diagnosis: toxic mastitis or metritis, botulism (12.69), periparturient hemorrhage, severe hind-limb trauma (7.90), bilateral obturator paralysis (7.91).

Management: slow i.v. injection of 400 mL of 40% calcium borogluconate, possibly with additional magnesium and phosphorus. Calcium may also be given by s.c. injection. Prevention includes avoidance of over-fat cows at calving, and dietary management during the transition period. Avoid lush high-potassium and high-calcium rations such as grazing, and feed long-fiber roughage and diets which have an appropriate cation:anion balance.

Nervous acetonemia (ketosis, "slow fever")

Nervous acetonemia is an intoxication by circulating ketone bodies and is associated with an energy deficit in early lactation. Typical clinical signs are anorexia and lethargy (hence "slow fever"), depressed yields, and constipation, although some cases develop nervous signs such as compulsive licking, salivation, biting flanks (as seen in this 5-year-old Holstein in 9.8), or even maniacal behavior. This cow was difficult to get in the parlor for milking. Six hours later her frantic licking of udder and forelegs resulted in bleeding. The cow rapidly responded to dextrose and corticosteroids.

Differential diagnosis: hypomagnesemia (9.4, 9.5), BSE (9.36–9.38), listeriosis (9.11, 9.12).

Management: avoid over-fat cows at calving. Provide suitable transition rations (see "Hypocalcemia", above), and palatable high-energy feed in early lactation.

Fatty liver syndrome (fat cow syndrome)

Definition: a condition of anorexia, ketonuria, and hepatic dysfunction in over-fat cows at parturition, precipitated by other peripartum diseases and disturbed feed intake, especially in cows that are fed an energy-deficient diet after calving.

Clinical features: many cows show no specific clinical signs. More advanced cases develop anorexia and "stargazing", progressing to toxemia and terminal recumbency.

9

9.7. Hypocalcemic cow with head resting on flank

9.8. Nervous acetonemia (ketosis) showing compulsive licking and teat trauma in cow (Holstein, 5 years old)

9.9. Fatty liver syndrome showing massive fatty infiltration of liver

Massive fatty infiltration of the friable liver is seen in 9.9. The plastic glove in 9.10 demonstrates the severe yellow scour typical of toxemia, which proved fatal in this dairy cow.

Differential diagnosis: hypocalcemia (9.6, 9.7), mastitis, metritis, and other forms of toxemia.

Management: early cases may respond to i.v. glucose solutions, parenteral glucocorticoids, and bovine somatotrophin (if licensed). Advanced recumbent cases should be culled. Prevention is as for ketosis (p. 161).

Bacterial infections

Listeriosis ("circling disease")

Definition: infectious disease caused by *Listeria monocytogenes*, resulting in either a meningoencephalitic syndrome, neonatal septicemia, or abortion.

Clinical features: the meningoencephalitic form produces pyrexia, dullness, blindness, head-pressing, and a unilateral facial nerve paralysis, leading to prolapse of the tongue (9.11) and drooping of the ears. Compulsive circling toward the affected side (9.12) is also often seen,

9.10. Yellow scour, typical of toxemia

9.11. Listeriosis with prolapsed tongue and drooping ears

and abortions may occur, but they are usually not concurrent with nervous signs. Note the typical paralyzed eyelids and resulting development of keratitis sicca in both 9.11 and 9.12. In 2–4-day-old calves septicemia leads to sudden death. *Listeria* can be isolated from many organs at autopsy. The organism is ubiquitous, being found in the environment and in most wildlife. Disease may be associated with cold weather and silage feeding.

Differential diagnosis: rabies (9.33), acute lead poisoning (13.29), CCN (9.1), BSE (9.36), botulism (12.69), bacterial meningitis (9.22), viral encephalitis, pituitary abscess (9.18).

Management: early cases may respond to aggressive penicillin therapy, with NSAIDs in initial stages. *Listeria* is more prevalent in high-pH silage and in moldy silage, so prevention is based on silage management. Preventive parenteral penicillin at birth may reduce deaths from neonatal septicemia.

Otitis externa

Definition: inflammation of the external ear canal characterized clinically by head-shaking, pawing at the ear and intermittent deviation of the head, pain, and

9.12. Listeriosis showing compulsive circling and keratitis sicca

9.13. Otitis externa with purulent exudate

aural discharge. The etiology may involve arthropod parasites, foreign bodies, or systemic infections. *Rhabditis bovis* is a common cause in tropical countries.

Clinical features: in the 2-month-old Holstein calf (9.13) the ear canal shows a superficial moist, red dermatitis with a purulent exudate. This resolved with topical and parenteral antibiotic therapy.

Differential diagnosis: otitis media (9.14, 9.15), listeriosis (9.11), meningitis (9.22), CCN (9.1).

Management: topical ivermectin, broad-spectrum antibiotics, and local cleansing.

Middle ear infection (otitis media)

Clinical features: in middle ear infections, the head is typically held to one side, as in the calf in 9.14 and the Friesian cow in 9.15. However, the cow remained alert, continued feeding, and was not pyrexic. Note the base-wide stance to maintain balance. *Pasteurella* spp., *Mycoplasma bovis* and other respiratory bacterial pathogens are often involved, and an increased incidence is often seen concurrent with outbreaks of respiratory disease.

Differential diagnosis: listeriosis (9.11), meningitis (9.22), otitis externa (9.13).

Management: some improvement is seen with parenteral antibiotics, but many cases continue to thrive, apparently unaffected by the head tilt. Prevention involves control of respiratory infections.

Facial nerve paralysis

Clinical features: in 9.16 the ear, upper eyelid, and muzzle are drooping. In this bull the cause was unknown, but possible etiology includes trauma, middle ear disease, listeriosis, and other brain infections.

Differential diagnosis: includes botulism (12.69), rabies (9.33), listeriosis (9.11).

9.14. Otitis media in calf

9

9.15. Otitis media: wide-based stance and tilted head in cow

9.16. Facial nerve paralysis involving ear, upper eyelid, and muzzle

Brain abscess

Clinical features: the Ayrshire cow in 9.17 looks apprehensive, holds her head to one side, and is unable to stand on her front legs. An abscess (A) was seen in the base of the brain on autopsy (9.18). A common location for such abscesses is the pituitary fossa. Pituitary abscessation is recognized clinically in cattle as a characteristic initial inability to close the jaws, prolapse of the tongue (9.19) with resulting drooling of saliva, followed by progressive loss of balance, recumbency, and death as in this Charolais bull which had been dehorned, leading to a

9.18. Brain abscess (A) at autopsy of cow in 9.17

septic frontal sinusitis. Autopsy (9.20) revealed abscessation (A) in the rete mirabile of the pituitary gland.

Differential diagnosis: listeriosis, thromboencephalomyelitis, acute lead poisoning, viral encephalitis, other space-occupying brain lesions.

Management: individual treatment is usually unsuccessful. Prevention depends on control of foci of bacteremia such as lameness, mastitis, and respiratory infections.

Meningitis/meningoencephalitis

Definition: a pathological inflammation of the meninges of variable etiology.

Clinical features: meningitis produces a range of clinical signs. Some calves have difficulty in standing and

9.17. Brain abscess: unable to stand on forelegs, abnormal head and neck posture in cow (Ayrshire)

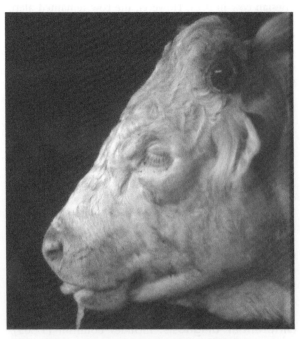

9.19. Pituitary abscess in bull, head view (France)

9.20. Pituitary abscess at brain autopsy (France)

walking, as in this 4-week-old Holstein heifer (9.21), which collapsed in the forequarters, and shortly afterwards went into extensor rigidity. The calf in 9.22 is leaning and pushing its head against the wall, its pupils are dilated, and it is frothing at the mouth. Some calves (9.23) are recumbent and dull, with drooping ears and eyelids, giving the appearance of an intense headache. The calf in 9.23 also had a hypopyon (see p. 152) which resolved surprisingly rapidly following treatment. Hypopyon is also just evident in 9.22. A more extreme case developed extensor spasm (9.24) and opisthotonos (9.25), but recovered. Adult cattle can also be affected with similar signs. 9.26 shows a typically congested brain at autopsy. A range of organisms may be involved including *Streptococci*, *Histophilus*, *Pasteurella*, and *Listeria*.

Differential diagnosis: rabies (9.33, 9.34), brain abscess (9.17), acute lead poisoning (13.29), infectious thromboembolic meningoencephalitis (9.27). CSF examination is important in differential diagnosis.

9.22. Meningitis: calf leaning against wall, dilated pupils, frothing

9.23. Meningitis: recumbent dull calf with drooping ears and eyelids

9.21. Meningitis: abnormal foreleg posture in heifer (Holstein, 4 weeks old)

9.24. Meningitis: extensor spasm and opisthotonus in calf

9

9.25. Meningitis: opisthotonus in calf of 9.24 (close-up)

9.27. Histophilosis (TEME, TME): depression and salivation in bull (Charolais) (Germany)

Histophilus somni disease complex (TEME, ITEME), thrombotic meningoencephalitis (TME), (histophilosis)

Definition: an acute, often fatal, septicemic disease involving one or multiple body systems, caused by *Histophilus somni*.

Clinical features: it is seen primarily in North American feedlot cattle but has also been reported in Europe and Israel. The correct terminology is disputed. TME (TEME, ITEME) is sudden in onset, occurring initially with marked pyrexia. Affected animals are dull and severely depressed, as in the Charolais bull in 9.27. Note the salivation, drooping ears and eyelids. Recumbency and death may follow within a few hours. Blindness from retinal hemorrhages with gray foci of retinal necrosis and edema are early features. Marked cerebral edema, congestion, and hemorrhage are seen in a ventral view of the brain (9.28) at autopsy, with congestion of the gray matter, cerebral hemorrhages (in the lateral ventricles), meningitis, and discolored cerebrospinal fluid (CSF). *H. somni* alone can cause a suppurative bronchopneumonia with severe cranioventral changes (9.29), or it may be involved in shipping fever or pasteurellosis. The

9.28. Histophilosis: brain showing marked edema and hemorrhage

9.26. Meningitis: congested meninges and brain at autopsy (USA)

9.29. Histophilosis: lungs showing severe cranioventral changes (USA)

9

pathogen can be cultured from many organs including synovia, CSF, pleural cavity, and myocardium.

Differential diagnosis: cerebrocortical necrosis (9.1, 9.3), hypovitaminosis A, acute lead poisoning (13.29), listeriosis (9.11, 9.12), pasteurellosis (5.10), rabies (9.33, 9.34).

Management: sick animals should be isolated and immediately given antibiotic therapy. Cattle which become recumbent with TME infection rarely recover, despite intensive care. Attempts to develop an effective preventive program with bacterins of *H. somni* have generally been unsuccessful in North America. Mass medication with longacting tetracycline on arrival in feedlots did not reduce mortality from *H. somni*, but has reduced the incidence of subsequent respiratory disease.

Coenurus cerebralis (coenurosis, "gid")

Etiology: *Coenurus cerebralis* is the intermediate stage (metacestode) of the canine tapeworm, *Taenia multiceps*. Although common in sheep, it occasionally encysts in cattle brains, producing a slow, progressive nervous disease.

Clinical features: starting with blindness, headpressing, sleepiness, and aimless wandering, affected animals eventually become recumbent over a period of 1–4 months. The Hereford cross heifer (9.30), unable to stand, has its eyes closed and head extended, believed typical of a headache. The cyst often lies immediately beneath the frontal bone, and can be removed surgically from the external surface of the cerebral hemispheres (9.31). This animal made a full recovery.

Management: correct carcass disposal to avoid dogs becoming infected with tapeworms. Regular 3-monthly treatment of all farm dogs and others in contact with livestock.

9.31. Coenurus cerebralis: removal of cyst from brain

Viral infections

Rabies

Definition: rabies is a rhabdoviral infection that produces a fatal encephalomyelitis in all warm-blooded animal species, including humans.

Clinical features: dogs, cats, and wild carnivores (e.g., foxes, raccoons, coyotes) are primarily affected. Carrier animals transmit infective saliva to cattle by biting, e.g., the vampire bat shown feeding from a cow in Brazil in 9.32 was later found to harbor the rabies virus. The virus then passes to the brain via peripheral nerves (ascending paralysis), hence the variation in incubation period depending on the site of injury. Initially seen simply as a change in behavior, early cases progress to show salivation, apprehension, bellowing (9.33), and knuckling of the hind fetlocks. Some cattle have marked tenesmus (9.34). This may lead directly to paralysis and death, although in the more classic "furious" form of rabies, with characteristic bellowing, aggression sometimes occurs in cattle. Pending euthanasia in the tropics a steer

9.30. Coenurus cerebralis infection ("gid") in recumbent steer with extended head (Hereford cross)

9.32. Rabies: vampire bat feeding from cow, later rabies positive (Brazil)

9.33. Rabies: bellowing steer, shackled for restraint

9.35. Aujeszky's disease (pseudorabies): apprehension, salivation, and self-inflicted injury from pruritus

may be shackled for restraint (9.33) due to the lack of isolation facilities.

Differential diagnosis: bacterial meningitis (9.22), brain abscess (9.17), listeriosis (9.11), botulism (12.70), Aujeszky's disease (9.35), hypomagnesemia (9.4, 9.5), nervous ketosis (9.8).

Management: countries free of rabies maintain strict quarantine measures for dogs and cats entering from abroad. Many other countries have active eradication campaigns and a compulsory vaccination policy for certain domestic species.

9.34. Rabies: marked tenesmus (Germany)

Aujeszky's disease (pseudorabies, "mad itch")

Definition: caused by porcine herpesvirus (SuHV-1), infection is occasionally acquired from pigs and causes a progressive and fatal disease with a characteristic frenzied scratching and marked excitement.

Clinical features: although primarily a herpes infection of pigs, other species, including cattle, can sporadically develop a meningoencephalitis that is usually fatal within 48 hours. Apprehension, licking, trembling, and salivation (9.35) are early signs, typically followed by an intense pruritus, marked excitement, paralysis, convulsions and death. The grossly swollen eyelids in 9.35 are the result of intense rubbing to relieve the pruritus.

Differential diagnosis: nervous acetonemia (9.8), rabies (9.33, 9.34), PPH (9.39), acute lead poisoning (13.29).

Management: this disease is notifiable. Some countries practice vaccination of cattle which are in close contact with potentially infected pigs.

Bovine spongiform encephalopathy (BSE)

Definition: BSE is a progressive nonfebrile, fatal brain degenerative condition. The full etiology is not yet understood, but the current theory is that it is an infectious disease caused by ingestion of an agent ("prion"), which may be present in ruminant-derived concentrate feed which is similar to but not necessarily identical to the

9.36. Bovine spongiform encephalopathy (BSE) with weight loss and abnormal gait

9.38. BSE: recumbent cow in "dog-sitting" posture, excitable

scrapie agent in sheep. The worldwide political and economic effects of BSE have been enormous.

Clinical features: cows that are between 3 and 6 years old are primarily affected by bovine spongiform encephalopathy. Occasional cases occur in bulls, and cases are more common in dairy than beef cows because the former are more likely to have been given concentrates as calves. Clinical signs include weight loss (9.36), an unsteady, stiff-legged gait, especially in the hind legs, and behavioral changes such as teeth grinding, excessive licking of the muzzle, muscle twitching, nervousness, over-reaction to stimuli such as a hand-clap, and occasionally aggression. Severe posterior ataxia and, eventually, recumbency develop after a period of days to months. The change in gait is difficult to portray in a photograph. The Friesian cow in 9.37 is typically in poor bodily condition, with arched back, raised tail, stiffness of hind legs, and her base-wide stance is an attempt to maintain balance in walking. She was difficult, indeed almost dangerous, to handle. Recumbent cases (9.38) often adopt a characteristic dog-sitting posture. Typical microscopic spongiform changes were seen in the brain at autopsy.

First seen in 1986, BSE was originally largely confined to the UK, with many fewer cases seen in Ireland and Switzerland. From the mid 1990s onwards, several hundred cases have been diagnosed in Portugal, France, Germany, and other European countries. Susceptibility to infection is possibly inherited, and maternal transmission via placenta or colostrum may occur. The disease is notifiable worldwide due to its possible association with the human form of new variant Creutzfeldt–Jakob disease (nvCJD). In the 10 years to 2010 the incidence has been steadily reduced.

Differential diagnosis: rabies (9.33, 9.34), Aujeszky's disease (9.35), listeriosis (9.11, 9.12), meningitis (9.21–9.26), brain abscess (9.17, 9.18), hypomagnesemia (9.4, 9.5).

Management: following notification, suspect cases are euthanized on the farm, and the brain is examined for diagnostic changes. Antemortem tests are currently under trial. In the UK only about 85% of clinically suspect animals prove to be positive. Control is based on the destruction of all potentially infected and clinically suspect cases, and by the total elimination of mammalian protein from ruminant feeds.

Miscellaneous disorders

Pruritus-pyrexia-hemorrhagica (PPH)

Definition: a rare, noninfectious disorder of adult cattle of uncertain etiology, causing an intense pruritus and variable other systemic signs.

Clinical features: in PPH, raised plaques of skin on the head (9.39), neck, tail, and udder may initially resemble ringworm (3.25, 3.26), but are intensely pruritic. More severe cases are pyrexic, anorexic, and pass blood from the mouth, nose, and rectum. The cause is unknown, but a fungal toxin, citronin, produced by *Penicillium* and *Aspergillus* molds and sweet vernal grass have both been

9.37. BSE: arched back, raised tail and stiff gait (Friesian, 5 years old)

9

9.39. Pruritus-pyrexia-hemorrhagica (PPH) with raised skin plaques on head

implicated. At autopsy intense hemorrhage is seen throughout the carcass including the heart, and also white, necrotic renal foci.

Differential diagnosis: Aujeszky's disease (9.35), mange (3.11), nervous ketosis (9.8), winter dysentery, especially the hemorrhagic form (4.19), ringworm (3.25).

Salt-craving pica

Prolonged deficient diets lead to an intense craving for salt. Affected animals will often lick and bite any object (pica), and may avidly attack salt blocks (9.40). Milk production, food intake, growth, and fertility may be depressed.

Lightning strike

Clinical features: animals that have been struck by lightning are typically found beside a hedge, a wire fence (9.41), or under a tree. The tree may show evidence of lightning damage. Trees that have shallow-spreading root systems are particularly dangerous, especially if the ground is damp or has underground drains. Dead animals may be found with fresh food in the mouth and scorch marks of burned hair on the coat, especially the legs (9.42). Removal of the hide reveals extensive bleeding due to rupture of the subcutaneous blood vessels (9.43). Mildly affected animals may recover after a variable period of time.

Differential diagnosis (of sudden death): hypomagnesemia (9.4), bloat (4.61), pulmonary thromboembolism (5.31–5.34), cardiac failure (see Chapter 6), anthrax (12.63).

9

9.40. Salt-craving pica: attraction of salt block (USA)

9.41. Lightning strike: fatalities along a wire fence

9.42. Lightning strike: burned hair, scorch marks

Electrocution

Clinical features: electrocution is quite commonly seen in cattle, partly owing to an inherent susceptibility, but also because they are more often exposed in milking parlors (9.44). Clinical signs vary from being stunned, with resulting nasal, oral, and ocular bleeding, to death (as in the cows in 9.44), also with profuse bleeding. Death is due to ventricular fibrillation and respiratory arrest. Exposure to lower levels of high-amperage electric current produces a variety of nervous and behavioral changes, depending on the voltage intensity. "Stray electricity", due to poor earthing, can be a problem in milking parlors, leading to poor milk let-down, and/or nervous cows liable frequently to kick off the cluster.

Management: regular servicing and improved maintenance of all electrical farm appliances is essential, and especially necessary in and around the milking parlor.

9.44. Electrocution: two fatalities in milking parlor with generalized bleeding

9.43. Lightning strike: extensive subcutaneous hemorrhage

9

Chapter 10

Urinogenital disorders

Introduction

This chapter is divided into disorders of the urinary tract, then of the male genital tract, and finally of the female genital tract. A short introduction to each group is given.

Urinary tract

Introduction

The main infectious and bacterial diseases of the bovine urinary tract are pyelonephritis and leptospirosis. Urolithiasis is a multifactorial urinary problem resulting from metabolic and nutritional disorders. Finally, amyloidosis, although an uncommon sporadic disease of adult cattle, requires differentiation from pyelonephritis.

Conditions with secondary renal pathology include pruritus-pyrexia-hemorrhagica (PPH) (9.39), oak (acorn) poisoning (13.6, 13.7), renal infarction secondary to caudal vena caval thrombosis (5.33), babesiosis (redwater, 12.39–12.43), and the many causes of bacteremia and septicemia.

Pyelonephritis

Definition: a bacterial infection (usually *Corynebacterium renale*) of the kidney and renal pelvis, pyelonephritis usually ascends from the vagina and vulva.

Clinical features: although worldwide in distribution, cases of pyelonephritis are sporadic only and overall incidence is low. Most often seen in the first 3 months postpartum, it may result from contact with infected urine or from a genital tract infection. Most infections start in the winter housing period when cow-to-cow contact increases. Affected cows are pyrexic, lose weight, show polyuria, hematuria or pyuria, and may develop a dry, brownish discoloration of the coat, often with urine staining over the tail and perineum which resembles cystitis (10.14). Rectal palpation may reveal a thickened ureter or enlarged (left) kidney. An 18-month-old Limousin heifer (10.1), ill for several days, showed at autopsy a granular renal cortex with areas of recent hemorrhage. In addition, several small discrete renal abscesses are evident, one of which has burst.

Severe chronic pyelonephritis is illustrated in 10.2 where the left kidney is contracted and pale, and the right kidney is enlarged and appears granular. Both ureters, particularly the left, are thickened as they contain pus and cellular debris (pyoureter).

Other cases of pyelonephritis have multiple caseous and purulent centers, primarily in the renal medulla which may be appreciated on rectal palpation.

In a case of chronic pyelonephritis (10.3) calculi (A) are present in the renal calyces, further calculi are in a thickened fibrotic ureter, and the bladder mucosa contains multiple petechiae (B).

Diagnosis is usually made on gross appearance of a urine sample, urine staining of the tail and perineum, and rectal palpation of the bladder and kidneys. Pyelonephritis and cystitis may coexist.

Differential diagnosis: urolithiasis, intestinal obstruction (in acute pyelonephritis), cystitis (10.14).

Management: early cases may respond to aggressive parenteral antibiotics for 7–10 days (e.g., amoxicillin, potentiated sulfonamides). Affected animals are best isolated. Advanced cases should be culled.

Leptospirosis

Definition: an infectious disease of both adult and young cattle with different clinical syndromes caused by the spirochete *Leptospira*.

10.1. Chronic pyelonephritis in heifer (Limousin, 18 months old)

10.4. Leptospirosis: dark, swollen kidneys suggestive of hemolytic crisis

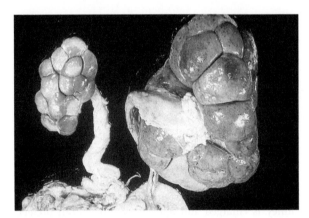

10.2. Severe chronic pyelonephritis and thickened ureters

Clinical features: in adults the main effects of *Leptospira interrogans* serovar *pomona* or *hardjo* infection are multiple abortions (see 10.86 for a fetus from a possible leptospiral abortion), stillbirths, loss of milk production, and reduced fertility. In calves *L. pomona* causes an acute septicemia with hemoglobinuria, jaundice, anemia, and possibly death. Dark, swollen kidneys (10.4) are usually indicative of a hemolytic crisis. Recovered cattle show little more than ill-defined, grayish, cortical spots, indicative of a focal interstitial nephritis. The spirochetes

may be seen under dark field microscopy of urine, but confirmation of diagnosis otherwise depends on serology or histopathology.

Differential diagnosis: babesiosis (12.39–12.43), anaplasmosis (12.44–12.47), rape and kale poisoning (13.10), postparturient hemoglobinuria, bacillary hemoglobinuria. Note the completely different appearances of the kidney in pyelonephritis (10.2) and amyloidosis (10.13).

Management: early clinical cases of *L. pomona* in adults with a hemolytic crisis may respond to tetracyclines. Blood transfusions may be additionally useful in acute syndromes in the calf. In early stages of a herd outbreak, further abortions may be avoided by prompt vaccination and antibiotic therapy of the entire herd.

Prevention: annual vaccination and rearing in confinement. *L. hardjo* control is difficult except in herds where only sporadic cases (abortion) are seen, when infected carrier cows may be culled. All new purchased cattle should be tested and only negative cattle retained. Whole herd vaccination has the risk of persistent renal *hardjo* carriers.

Urolithiasis

Definition: formation of calculi within the urinary tract.

Etiology: urolithiasis has a multifactorial etiology including dietary mineral imbalance, a relatively reduced fluid intake, high concentrate intake, and castration. The condition begins with microcalculus formation in the kidneys (10.3), and clinical problems arise when the calculi grow to a sufficient size to obstruct the urethra. The clinical syndrome is confined to the male (castrate or entire) where the urethral diameter is smaller.

Clinical features: early cases are dull, anorexic, and walk stiffly. If grown sufficiently, rectal examination may reveal an enlarged and painful bladder. Diagnosis is

10.3. Chronic pyelonephritis and renal calculi

10.5. Urolithiasis: struvite crystals on preputial hairs

10.7. Urolithiasis: ruptured urethra and subcutaneous swelling containing urine

10.8. Urolithiasis: scrotal view of swelling following urethral rupture

made on the basis of changes in the preputial region. Although preputial crystals (often struvite, i.e., magnesium-ammonium-phosphate hexahydrate) appear in many calves (10.5), relatively few will develop signs of obstruction, which tends to occur in or just proximal to the sigmoid flexure, or in the distal portion of the penis. An intraoperative view (10.6) of the perineal region shows the dilated urethra proximal to the sigmoid flexure and the obstructing calculus. Continuing complete urethral obstruction results in either bladder or, more commonly, urethral rupture. The crossbred Charolais male in (10.7) has a large subcutaneous swelling containing urine as a result of urethral rupture in the sigmoid region. The swelling extends forward from the sigmoid to the preputial orifice, where dry preputial hairs are covered with crystals. A rear view (10.8) shows gross enlargement of the scrotum, especially at the neck, early bruising, and a superficial fluid ooze, all caused by accumulated urine. In occasional cases the swelling is discretely localized to the peripreputial area. In contrast, in a severe and advanced case the Friesian steer (10.9) had such severe swelling that ischemic necrosis has caused an extensive skin slough overlying the penis.

In another Hereford steer (10.10) it is the bladder rather than the urethra that has ruptured as a result of urethral obstruction. Urine has gathered in the ventral abdominal cavity, causing a progressive swelling and distension of the flanks (uroperitoneum).

Autopsy examination of a 6-year-old Shorthorn bull that died as a result of severe uremia following bladder rupture and uroperitoneum reveals a congested and hemorrhagic bladder mucosa (10.11). Numerous calculi

10

10.6. Urolithiasis: obstructing calculus in urethra at ischial arch at surgery

10.9. Urolithiasis: ventral skin slough following urine extravasation in steer (Friesian)

10.10. Urolithiasis: bladder and uroperitoneum in steer (Hereford)

(2–7 mm diameter) and fibrin are seen on the mucosal surface. The peritoneum tends to be diffusely inflamed, but the changes are less severe than those following septic reticuloperitonitis (4.90, 4.91). Urolithiasis frequently accompanies cases of severe pyelonephritis (10.1–10.3).

Differential diagnosis: in a mature bull this includes penile hematoma (10.23) or abscess formation, or, in a younger animal, urethral rupture due to faulty application of a bloodless castrator (Burdizzo) some days previously (see 10.36). Differentials for cases with ventral abdominal swelling not localized to the penis and prepuce include ascites (4.92), intestinal obstruction (4.88), and generalized peritonitis with massive exudation (4.91). Other differential diagnoses include cystitis (10.14), severe balanoposthitis, and severe preputial frostbite.

Management: cases of severe uremia will not pass meat inspection, so if the bladder and urethra are intact, antispasmodics may be tried for a limited period. If blockage persists, a perineal urethrotomy dorsal to the scrotum (10.6) is a salvage procedure. Urine scald and urethrostomal stricture may be subsequent problems. An alternative treatment is to make several skin incisions over the urine-filled area to facilitate drainage, and then to allow continued urine flow through the skin. Rarely, a palpable single calculus can be removed by surgery. Fattening steers with distal urethral rupture and skin slough can also be salvaged to fatten.

Prevention: correction of calcium : phosphorus ratio in ration (about 2 : 1), avoidance of excessive magnesium. Many calf rations now include ammonium chloride as a urinary acidifier. Provision of supplementary salt in concentrate feed (2–5%) which drastically increases fluid intake and dilutes urine, therefore ensure easy access to fresh drinking water. Control possible primary cystitis (see below).

Amyloidosis

Definition: extracellular deposition of abnormal almost insoluble protein, amyloid, in various tissues is a sporadic disease. Reactive amyloidosis is derived from excessive serum amyloid A (SAA) produced following chronic antigenic stimulation. More common is idiopathic (secondary) amyloidosis associated with chronic suppurative conditions.

Clinical features: the marked presternal edema in the 3-year-old Limousin bull in 10.12 was caused by severe bilateral renal amyloidosis, which is characterized by polyuria and massive proteinuria leading to pronounced hypoproteinemia.

In a chronic suppurative condition the bull's kidney in 10.13 is markedly enlarged, pale, waxy, and granular in comparison with the normal kidney above it. This degree of enlargement should be detectable on rectal palpation.

Differential diagnosis: diagnosis is difficult, especially in the presence of coexisting disease, including pyelonephritis.

10.11. Urolithiasis: bladder rupture with mucosa showing calculi and hemorrhage in bull (Shorthorn, 6 years old)

10.12. Amyloidosis: presternal edema from renal amyloidosis in bull (Limousin, 3 years old)

10.13. Amyloidosis: enlarged, pale amyloid kidney; normal kidney above

Management: amyloidosis is incurable, and cannot be prevented.

Cystitis

Definition: inflammation of the bladder which may be associated with pyelonephritis, urolithiasis, or be idiopathic or mechanical in origin, e.g. following vaginal trauma at service.

Clinical features: the 6-month-old heifer in 10.14 passed urine frequently and in small amounts. The perineal region had a foul odor of stale urine and shows excoriation as a result of urine dribbling. The tail is slightly elevated, indicative of urinary tenesmus. A thickened bladder wall is often detectable on rectal examination of older animals.

10.14. Cystitis: perineal excoriation following urine dribbling in heifer (Friesian, 6 months old)

Differential diagnosis: urinalysis will differentiate pyelonephritis and urolithiasis.

Management: aggressive parenteral amoxicillin or trimethoprim-sulfa drugs is usually effective in uncomplicated cases.

Male genital tract

10

Introduction

The anatomical separation of parts of the male genital tract, and their common development with parts of the urinary tract, makes integration of this section difficult. It starts with congenital conditions, and continues with abnormalities affecting the penis, prepuce, scrotum, and, finally, the epididymis and seminal vesicles. Some congenital anomalies (e.g., persistent frenulum, cryptorchidism, and testicular hypoplasia)

10.15. Persistent preputial frenulum with penile deviation

10.16. Persistent frenulum

may not become apparent until breeding age (1–2 years old).

Congenital male abnormalities

Pseudohermaphrodite (freemartin)

Definition: an individual with gonads of one sex but with contradictions in the morphological criteria of sex.

Clinical features: the condition is rare. The animal may be mistaken for female at birth owing to the origin of the urine flow. The freemartin condition is illustrated in 10.40–10.42.

Persistent penile preputial frenulum

Definition: persistence of or incomplete separation of the penis and prepuce along the ventral raphé during the first year.

Clinical features: in 10.15 the penile body remains attached to the prepuce by a fine, longitudinal band of connective tissue (A). Persistent penile frenulum causing penile deviation is a congenital anomaly, but signs, such as ventral penile deviation or a failure of complete protrusion, are usually first seen at attempted intromission. In some breeds it is inherited, and surgically corrected bulls should not be used to sire replacement breeding stock. A 2-year-old Angus bull (10.16) presented for a fertility check following recent purchase, had a long-standing penile-preputial adhesion (contrast 10.15). The bull was returned to the seller. Surgical correction was considered unethical.

Testicular hypoplasia with cryptorchidism

The left testicle is descended and of normal size in the Friesian calf in 10.17. The right testicle, which is small and incompletely descended, is in the scrotal neck.

10.17. Cryptorchidism in hypoplastic right testicle of calf (Friesian)

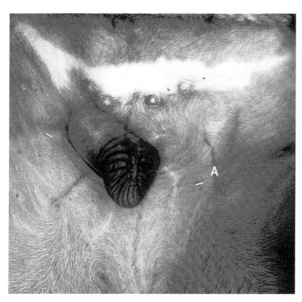

10.18. Cryptorchidism: left testicle is in inguinum (A)

Cryptorchidism

Definition: a condition characterized by incomplete development of one or both testes, including small size and incomplete descent.

Clinical features: bovine cryptorchidism is a not infrequent finding in batches of calves presented for castration. All breeds are affected although there is also a possible association with the polled character. In the 4-week-old Hereford cross calf in 10.18, the normal right testicle is in the scrotal sac, but the left testicle is in an inguinal position (A). The misplaced gonad has deviated from the normal course of descent and may be termed an "ectopic testicle." The undescended testicle is invariably considerably smaller, and when incised the seminiferous tissue is very pale in color.

Management: unless the animal is clearly identified, it is not safe to remove only the scrotal testicle because the undescended testicle may descend into the scrotum later in life, and potentially lead to unwanted pregnancies. Management options include leaving both testicles and re-examining the animal a few months later; surgically to remove the undescended testicle through the inguinal skin (which was the option chosen for 10.18); or to fatten the young bull for beef.

Penile conditions

Fibropapilloma ("wart")

Definition: a benign tumor of epithelial and connective tissue caused by a species-specific papovavirus.

Clinical features: the 2-year-old Friesian bull in 10.19 has several highly vascular, ulcerated masses attached to

10.19. Penile fibropapilloma on glans of bull (Friesian, 2 years old)

the glans penis. Caudal to the large mass is a smaller, more sessile fibropapilloma. These are typical sites for such multiple, proliferating masses, which are infectious, and relatively common in groups of young bulls confined in a small area.

Management: small tumors slowly regress , and like teat warts have resolved by 2–3 years of age. Large masses may cause persistent penile protrusion and require removal (e.g., by ligation) or retention within the prepuce by a purse-string suture, which was the option chosen for 10.19. 10.20 shows the same bull 4 months later and soon afterwards he was used for service. In some cases healing is accompanied by scarring and distortion

10

10.20. Penile fibropapilloma bull of fig 10.19 after 4 months

10.21. Penile deviation ("corkscrew penis") in bull (Charolais, 2 years old)

of the penile tunic, resulting in penile deviation and failure of intromission.

Spiral deviation of penis ("corkscrew penis")

Definition: spiral deviation is due to slipping of the dorsal apical ligament of the penis and may occur intermittently.

Clinical features: a spiral or corkscrew penile conformation is a normal occurrence at ejaculation in the vagina, but premature corkscrewing may be severe enough to prevent intromission. The first case (10.21), a 2-year-old Charolais, shows a 90° ventral curvature. The second case (10.22) clearly illustrates the spiraling effect, and the difficulty of intromission. In some bulls, an ulcer

10.22. Penile deviation with severe spiraling showing problem of intromission

10.23. Penile hematoma ("broken penis") with secondary penile prolapse in bull (Hereford)

on the glans penis indicates abrasion from repeated perineal contact. Rarely is the condition traumatic in origin.

Differential diagnosis: persistent penile frenulum in young bulls, scarring following fibropapillomata.

Management: surgical correction is possible, but ethical consideration is important if an inherited condition is suspected.

Penile and parapenile hematoma ("fracture of penis", "broken penis")

Definition and pathogenesis: a localized collection of blood involves the corpus cavernosum penis (CCP) and is almost always through the dorsal wall of the tunica, just distal to the sigmoid flexure. The tunica albuginea is ruptured, producing a prescrotal hematoma and edema. Rupture occurs at ejaculation, or, less commonly, at intromission when the fully engorged penis is suddenly bent beyond its physiological limits, for example, when the cow or heifer suddenly moves.

Clinical features: a discrete swelling is seen in the Hereford bull in 10.23, which also had a secondary prolapse of the penis. He cannot serve. The extent of the ruptured CCP is evident in the autopsy specimen of an affected penis (10.24) in which the sigmoid flexure (A)

10.24. Penile hematoma, showing ruptured corpus cavernosum penis at autopsy

10.25.   Penile trauma

10.26.   Preputial prolapse in bull (Brahman, 6 years old) (South Africa)

is just proximal to the mass. The black wire has been inserted into the urethra.

Differential diagnosis: parapenile abscess (10.27), urolithiasis (10.5–10.10).

Management: small lesions may resolve after 4–6 months' rest in isolation away from cycling females. When service is attempted, some bulls experience further bleeding. Some cases develop into parapenile abscesses, at which stage surgical correction (careful drainage and evacuation) is no longer useful.

External penile trauma

A Limousin bull running with a 400-cow dairy herd was presented with preputial bleeding post service. Rectal stimulation to give penile extrusion (10.25) showed that the distal penis had been totally severed and a portion of approximately 15–20 cm was missing. There is a secondary superficial infection of the residual stump. The bull showed no systemic signs but culling for meat was the only option.

Preputial conditions

Prolapsed prepuce (preputial eversion)

Definition: mucosa lining the preputial cavity prolapses through the preputial orifice.

Clinical features: preputial prolapse occurs as a breed characteristic in *Bos indicus*, e.g., Brahman and Santa Gertrudis, and in polled breeds which are liable to have comparatively weaker preputial muscles, although horned bulls may also be affected. Injury and infection are common causes. A partial preputial prolapse of comparatively recent onset is shown in a 6-year-old Brahman from South Africa (10.26). The mucosa has a granular appearance, with areas of superficial hemorrhage. More

severe cases are very prone to secondary trauma and edema.

Management: careful conservative medical management by cleansing, disinfection, and replacement of the prolapse and retention by a purse-string suture. Surgical resection is required in severe cases. More serious cases cannot initially be replaced and must be pressure-bandaged, with daily bandage changes, to reduce the size of the prolapse.

Preputial and penile abscess

Clinical features: in the 5-year-old Hereford bull in 10.27 the penis has been manually prolapsed. The hand holds the prepuce and penis just caudal to the point of attachment of the preputial mucosa (internal lamina) to the body of the penis, shown as a transverse fold. Pus oozes from a mucosal tear incurred when the penis was extended. Deep-red erectile tissue is evident in the defect. Below the wound, the mucosa is smooth and slightly pinkish-gray due to a further abscess pocket.

10

10.27.   Penile abscess in bull (Hereford, 5 years old)

10.28.   Penile and preputial prolapse in bull (Piedmontese)

Management: the prognosis is poor since effective and complete drainage of many abscesses in this area is difficult.

Posthitis and balanoposthitis

Definition: posthitis is an inflammation of the prepuce; balanoposthitis is an inflammation of both prepuce and penis.

Clinical features: the Piemontese bull in 10.28 developed a sudden prolapse of the prepuce and penis. Normal pink prepuce is visible at the skin junction. The central region of the prepuce is damaged (posthitis), the distal part of which forms a tight band around the penis, constricting the blood flow. The pink penis is congested and enlarged. The bull recovered well following conservative management to retain the prolapse within the prepuce for 5 weeks with a purse-string suture .

Some cases of balanoposthitis are due to genital IBR infection (10.29). This case of herpesvirus (BHV-1) balanoposthitis shows multiple pale vesicles, some of which are confluent, in the preputial mucosa. The reflection of the prepuce onto the penis is to the right. Other cases of

10.29.   Balanoposthitis due to IPVV infection, compare with fig 5.7.

10.30.   Inguinal hernia in bull (Sussex) (Zimbabwe)

balanoposthitis have a traumatic origin. See 5.7 on p. 85 for other details of IPVV.

Management: medical. Most cases resolve spontaneously. Some cases develop severe and extensive adhesions, and then have a poor prognosis.

Scrotal conditions

Inguinal hernia

Clinical features: there is a soft, reducible swelling in the inguinal region overlying the two rudimentary teats in this Sussex bull from Zimbabwe (10.30). Neither the scrotal neck nor the body is enlarged, showing that only the inguinal canal is involved. An inguinal hernia may contain omentum, or both omentum and small intestinal loops. Cattle have a genetic predisposition to inguinal hernia, inheritance being recessive.

Differential diagnosis: in overconditioned animals it can be difficult to differentiate fat deposits from a hernia. Abscessation is also possible.

Management: affected bulls should not be used to sire replacement stock.

Scrotal hernia

Definition: an inguinal hernia which has passed into the scrotum.

Clinical features: in 10.31 a 6-year-old Hereford bull shows an obvious swelling in the left side of the scrotal neck. It was soft, painless, and partially reducible. This scrotal hernia resulted in the production of very poor-quality semen due to local hyperthermia. The hernia had been acquired as a result of traumatic injury, and was not

10.31. Scrotal hernia in bull (Hereford, 6 years old) (USA)

congenital. Scrotal hernia is rare in cattle, and seldom results in intestinal strangulation.

Differential diagnosis: unilateral orchitis (10.32).

Management: cull, as surgery is difficult.

Orchitis

Definition: inflammation of a testis.

Clinical features: in 10.32 the scrotum of a 4-year-old Simmental bull shows enlargement of the right testis, which is more dependent than the left. Note that the scrotal neck is not swollen. The testis was painful and

10.33. Acute *Brucella* orchitis and periorchitis (A) with edema (B)

sensitive to touch. The etiology of this unilateral orchitis was probably traumatic, although various bacterial path- ogens, including *Brucella abortus, Mycobacterium bovis,* and *Arcanobacterium pyogenes,* have been implicated in other cases. In the acute *Brucella* orchitis illustrated in 10.33, the inflammatory reaction in the tunics and epididymis caused a severe periorchitis (pale areas, A), with early testicular necrosis as a result of testicular enlargement, and compression by the tunica albuginea. Ventrally, ede- matous fluid lies subcutaneously.

Differential   diagnosis: scrotal   hernia,   scrotal hematoma.

Management: antibiotic therapy may be used in early stages to prevent generalized effects, but recovered animals should be culled and not used for breeding.

Scrotal hematoma

Clinical features: Though here seen in a Holstein, scrotal hematoma is more common in beef bulls follow- ing trauma (10.34). The scrotum is swollen and tense but relatively painless. The testicle remains normal, despite the large volume of blood on the right side.

Differential   diagnosis: orchitis,   (10.32),   scrotal hernia (10.31).

Management: most cases resolve spontaneously.

Scirrhous cord

Definition: fibrotic infected enlarged stump of spermatic cord following castration, often with microabscessation.

10.32. Orchitis (right) in bull (Simmental, 4 years old) (South Africa)

10

10.34. Scrotal hematoma in bull (Holstein)

Clinical features: the scrotum is very swollen in the 4-month-old Friesian calf in 10.35. A dried blood clot lies over the ventral scrotal incision (castration). Exploration revealed an enlarged stump of the spermatic cord, which resulted from infection acquired at surgery. Immediate post-castration hemorrhage, with gross scrotal enlargement, is a major predisposing factor, and may result in abscess formation, pyrexia, and other systemic signs. Such wounds predispose calves to tetanus.

Management: in most calves provision of good drainage and flushing the scrotal hematoma or abscess,

10.36. Scrotal necrosis and gangrene following faulty use of bloodless castrator

cleansing of the stump, and systemic antibiotics for 5–7 days is effective. The prognosis will be less favorable if the spermatic cord is palpably swollen and painful where it enters the inguinal canal. In persisting problem cases amputation of the stump of cord including all areas of microabscessation may be needed.

Prevention: clean surgical technique and aftercare (e.g., clean straw).

Scrotal necrosis and gangrene

Clinical features: the Friesian calf in 10.36 has an irregular necrotic line at the scrotal neck, separating gangrenous from normal tissue. The reaction is a result of faulty application of a bloodless castrator (Burdizzo). A continuous, crushed line encircles the scrotal neck, cutting off the blood supply to the lower skin. The same effect is obtained when a rubber castration ring is placed around the scrotal neck, and all tissue distal to the ring undergoes atrophy. When this is done relatively late, i.e., after 1 week old, the reaction is much more severe. In the Friesian calf in 10.37 the ring was applied at 2 months. Welfare legislation makes this procedure illegal in many countries. Note the considerable swelling proximal to the ring, compared with the shriveled, dark, necrotic distal portion.

If a bloodless castrator is applied too high, the urethra may be accidentally crushed, leading to urethral rupture and a ventral, subcutaneous accumulation of urine similar to that following urethral calculus obstruction (10.9). Many countries have legal (statutory) upper limits on the age at which Burdizzo and rubber ring castration may be carried out.

Differential diagnosis: urolithiasis.

10.35. Scirrhous cord beneath scrotal incision in calf (Friesian, 4 months old)

Management: calves with proximal tissue swelling (10.37) should be given prophylactic antibiotics. Other cases may be left to slough naturally.

10.37. Scrotal necrosis following late application of rubber castration ring

Scrotal frostbite

Clinical features: moderate frostbite affected the bottom of the scrotum of a 2-year-old Simmental (10.38) following exposure to a temperature of −30°C in Saskatchewan, Canada, 2–8 weeks previously. The semen

10.38. Scrotal frostbite in bull (Simmental, 2 years old) (Canada)

10.39. Seminal vesiculitis showing cystic and hemorrhagic changes in left seminal vesicle at autopsy

quality was poor (<10% live cells). Most cases return to normal semen quality within 2–3 months.

Seminal vesiculitis

Clinical features: although the right seminal vesicle of the bull in 10.39 is normal and the ampulla has its lumen exposed, the left ampulla is absent and the left seminal vesicle shows cystic, hemorrhagic, and mild inflammatory changes (A). (B) is the pelvic urethra. Seminal vesiculitis causes a purulent, preputial discharge after service, or pus may be seen in semen collected for artificial insemination (AI). Common organisms include *Arcanobacterium pyogenes*, *Brucella*, and *Escherichia coli*. Young bulls are predominantly involved.

Diagnosis: seminal vesiculitis is diagnosed by rectal palpation and semen examination. Lack of symmetry, firmness, and pain are the significant findings.

Management: incurable.

10

Female genital tract

Introduction

Maintenance of optimum fertility is of major economic importance in both beef and dairy herds. A high lifetime output of milk and calves can be attained only if cows breed regularly, and considerable effort is expended on fertility examinations, health control, disease prevention, and optimal nutrition to achieve this. Much of this work cannot be adequately illustrated. Poor management techniques, e.g., poor heat detection, are best demonstrated by an analysis of herd breeding records, and are not discussed in this atlas. Mineral and trace element deficiencies may affect fertility by reducing conception rates or interrupting ovarian cycles, but again cannot be demonstrated pictorially.

Diseases and disorders of the female genital tract are numerous. This section starts with a description of female anatomical, congenital and developmental abnormalities, including cystic ovaries and neoplasia of the tract. The latter is comparatively rare. Dystocia is difficult to illustrate. Many conditions are diagnosed and corrected by intravaginal and intrauterine manipulation. Postpartum complications include vaginal wall rupture and hemorrhage, prolapse of parts of the genital tract (uterine prolapse is the most common) and metritis, endometritis, and pyometra, all of which are sequelae of dystocia, which in turn may be partly the result of poor bull selection. There is often a conflict of interest between the use of a large breed bull to produce valuable offspring and a small breed to facilitate easy parturition. Not all pregnancies reach term and the final section of the chapter illustrates some causes of abortion and premature calving.

Congenital abnormalities

Intersexuality and freemartinism result from placental fusion in early pregnancy. Segmental aplasia of the Müllerian duct system is inherited and leads to a range of abnormalities including white heifer disease (imperforate hymen). Ovarian agenesis, ovarian hypoplasia, and fallopian tube aplasia have all been reported, but they are rare and therefore not illustrated.

Freemartinism

Definition: a sterile female born twin with a male.

Clinical features: in cattle, over 90% of twin calves have fused placentae, with a common blood supply. 10.40

10.40. Twin fetuses showing fused placentae

10.41.   Freemartin calf with enlarged clitoris

shows how small the point of fusion may be. The heifer calf starts its development as a female, but, owing to the interchange of embryonic cells and hormones between the 30th and 40th days of pregnancy (i.e., before the stage of sexual dimorphism), many develop male characteristics. The freemartin is probably masculinized by the secretion from its own gonads. The Friesian animal in 10.41 has an enlarged clitoris, and excess hair is growing as a tuft from the ventral vulval commissure. On rectal examination, no internal genitalia could be palpated beyond the cervix. Testicles were present in the scrotum, the right side of which is enlarged. Varying degrees of hypoplasia and masculinization may be seen. 10.42 demonstrates hypoplasia of the anterior vagina (A), an absence of the cervix, vestigial ovaries (B), and testes (C) that are joined to the immature uterine horns by ducts.

Diagnosis: a short vaginal length, checked in 2–4-week old heifer calves using a test tube, confirms a freemartin, although by no means all calves with a normal vaginal

length are entire. Most cases are identified by rectal palpation of nonbreeding heifers, and by external genital changes. Blood-sampling for chromosome analysis is possible as a freemartin has white cells containing both XY and XX chromosomes.

Segmental uterine aplasia ("white heifer disease", imperforate hymen)

Definition: segmental uterine aplasia is a developmental defect of the Müllerian duct system, in which ovarian development allows normal estrus behavior, but the hymen is often persistent. Pregnancy may occur in mild cases, with the persistent hymen sometimes leading to dystocia.

Clinical features: in the advanced case shown in 10.43, the right uterine horn is aplastic, the residual portion (A) being dilated with cyclical fluid. This could be classified as uterus unicornis. The condition is due to a sex-linked recessive gene, but, despite its popular name of white heifer disease, it is not always related to coat color.

Double cervix (double os uteri externum)

Only the external cervical os is duplicated in this second example of a Müllerian duct defect (10.44). An endoscopic view (10.45) illustrates placental membranes, visible through the left (upper dark) os. This relatively common congenital condition leads to surprisingly few incidents of dystocia.

10

10.42.   Freemartin (specimen) with no cervix, small testes, and vestigial ovaries

10.43.   Segmental uterine aplasia (white heifer disease) with aplastic right uterine horn at autopsy

10.44. Double cervix at autopsy

Ovarian disorders

Cystic ovaries

Ovarian cysts arise from a failure of ovulation. The anovulatory follicle increases in size to produce a fluid-filled structure greater than 2.5 cm in diameter, and normal ovarian cycles are usually interrupted. Cysts are not incompatible with pregnancy, however, and abattoir studies show a surprising number of pregnant cows with cysts. Stress, mineral and trace element deficiencies, feeding for high milk yields, and heredity are among the suggested causes. Although classically subdivided into luteal and follicular cysts, there is probably a degree of interchange between the two forms. Many cysts resolve

10.45. Double cervix seen through endoscope showing dark placental membranes (Germany)

10.46. Luteal cyst in left ovary (thick-walled)

spontaneously, especially those occurring in early lactation, whilst others require treatment.

Luteal cyst

In 10.46 a single, large, spherical, thick-walled cyst is present in the left ovary. Luteal cysts secrete progesterone and may lead to prolonged anestrus. The right ovary contains an incised cystic corpus luteum.

Follicular cyst

In 10.47 the right ovary contains a large, thin-walled follicular cyst. Such cysts are invariably estrogenic and lead to irregular or prolonged estrus periods. Multilocular follicular cysts frequently occur. A corpus luteum, 5–7 days old, is present in the left ovary, suggesting that normal cyclicity can continue in the nonaffected ovary. Cows with unresolved follicular cysts may develop both a raised tail head as a result of relaxation of the pelvic ligaments

10.47. Follicular cyst in right ovary (thin-walled)

10

10.48. Raised tail head characteristic of persistent follicular cysts

10.50. Hydrosalpinx with massive fluid distension (A)

(10.48), and characteristic male behavioral changes, such as deep bellowing and pawing the ground.

Management: control predisposing factors. Treatment with prostaglandin, GnRH, or progesterone-releasing devices.

Bursal adhesions and hydrosalpinx

The bursa in 10.49 is tightly adherent to a large cyst in the right ovary, the oviduct (A) of which is distended with fluid (hydrosalpinx). The small visible portion (B) of the left oviduct is normal, and the left ovary contains a 3–5-day-old corpus luteum (C). Bursal adhesions and hydrosalpinx can both result from rough handling of the ovary during, for example, manual rupture of ovarian cysts and enucleation of corpora lutea.

Hydrosalpinx is more pronounced in the oviduct of 10.50, which is grossly distended with fluid (A) following a loss of patency. A small segment of normal duct (B) is visible on the bursa, as well as a 6–8-day-old corpus luteum on the ovary (C).

Management: adhesions alone do not necessarily result in infertility, as the fallopian tube may remain patent. Patency can be tested by intrauterine infusion of dye.

Female genital tract tumors

Incidence: granulosa cell tumors are by far the most common ovarian neoplasms, but fibromas, sarcomas, and carcinomas have been reported. Uterine fibromyomas, leiomyomas, and lymphosarcomas are rare, whilst fibropapillomas (polyps) of the vagina and cervix are not uncommon.

Ovarian granulosa cell tumor

Definition: ovarian stromal neoplasm developing in the solid granulosa cells surrounding the ovum in the developing Graafian follicle.

Clinical features: a large cystic neoplasm is seen in the right ovary in 10.51. Initially estrogen-secreting, such tumors cause nymphomania. Advanced cases undergo

10

10.49. Bursal adhesions on large right ovarian cyst

10.51. Ovarian granulosa cell tumor (right)

10.52. Uterine lymphosarcoma or lymphoma with multiple tan masses (USA)

luteinization, leading to anestrus or even masculinization. The incised uterine horn shows endometrial hyperplasia and mucometra.

Management: surgical ovariectomy is a simple procedure, although most cases would be culled.

Uterine lymphosarcoma (lymphoma)

Clinical features: usually seen as one of a number of sites for neoplasia in enzootic (adult) bovine leukosis (EBL), (12.80, 12.81), including heart, spinal canal (7.81), and liver, such uterine involvement (10.52) is easily appreciated on rectal palpation for pregnancy diagnosis. The mass is firm and smooth, and local lymphadenopathy (lumbar nodes) is usually appreciable. Autopsy reveals multiple nodules of soft tan tissue in the uterine wall (10.52). All the masses involve the uterine wall, which has been incised at two points to show the thickness.

Differential diagnosis: early stage pregnancy, other uterine tumors (10.53).

Management: early cull.

Uterine fibromyoma

Definition: benign tumor containing fibroid elements, or leiomyoma.

Clinical features: seen as a smooth mass involving much of the uterine wall (10.53), and easily palpable on rectal examination. This type of tumor does not necessarily interrupt pregnancy.

Hydrops allantois and hydrops amnii

Definition: excess fluid accumulating in the allantoic or amniotic sac, or both.

Clinical features: in hydrops allantois (hydrallantois) the lower abdomen is grossly and tightly distended bilaterally as a result of excess fluid accumulating in the uterus, usually in the allantoic sac (10.54). The condition develops in the seventh to ninth months of pregnancy, and is seen initially as a slowly progressive abdominal distention, with weight loss, inappetance, increasing dyspnea, difficulty in rising, and eventual recumbency. Fetal death may occur, and hydrops may result in the rupture of the prepubic tendon (3.71). Fluid volumes of up to 300 liters have been recorded (normal: 8–10 liters).

Differential diagnosis: twins or triplets, ascites (4.92), large abdominal tumor, other causes of weight loss.

Management: induce parturition with prostaglandin $F_{2\alpha}$ or an analog, or corticosteroids. Shock, uterine inertia, dystocia, and retained placenta are common

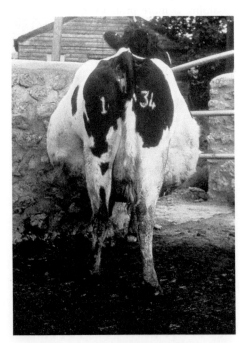

10.54. Hydrops allantois (hydrops amnii) with typical abdominal distension

10.53. Uterine fibromyoma

10

complications, which are frequently fatal. Slaughter without treatment is likely to result in carcass condemnation for edema and emaciation, while welfare considerations prohibit transport in many countries.

Dystocia

Definition: difficult parturition.

Etiology: dystocia in cattle may be due to twins, fetal postural defects, fetal monstrosities (e.g., anasarca (10.60) and schistosomus reflexus (1.10)), maternal problems (e.g., uterine torsion), and disproportion between fetal and maternal size. The latter is the most common cause, especially in heifers, and typically results from small, undersized heifers, or from inappropriate bull selection leading to an oversized fetus, or from excessive fat restricting the available space in the pelvic birth canal by overfeeding of the dam. The conditions illustrated in this section are chosen as examples. The list is by no means comprehensive.

Management: many management options are available, e.g., traction, manual fetal manipulation (for malpresentation), embryotomy, cesarian section, etc.

Prevention: correct sire selection and maternal nutrition.

Head only presentation

The case in 10.55 is not a longstanding dystocia, as the head is moist, of normal size, and has no tongue protrusion. The shoulders will be at the pelvic inlet, the forelimbs in the uterus.

Head and one leg presentation

In 10.56 a more longstanding case of dystocia ("leg back") is illustrated. The head is dry and swollen and the protruding tongue is edematous. The enlarged and edematous vulval lips may persist for 24–48 hours after parturition.

10.56. Dystocia: head and one leg presentation

Three legs and no head presented

The most common cause of this presentation (10.57) is the presence of twins, although other causes are possible. Note how three ropes have been applied, one on each leg and one on the head of the lower twin. The upper foot of the second twin needs to be repelled before delivery of the first calf.

Posterior presentation with fetal dorsoventral rotation

Initial observation of the calf's feet and fetlocks in 10.58 might suggest a case of anterior presentation, with lateral deviation of the head (head back). Closer inspection shows the hocks at the vulva, but the point of the hock (os calcis) is ventral. Rotation facilitated delivery of a live calf.

10

10.55. Dystocia: head only presentation

10.57. Dystocia: presentation of three legs; head, and one leg back (of twins)

10.58. Dystocia: posterior presentation with fetal rotation

Breech presentation (hip flexion)

In 10.59 only the tail is visible and there is no vulval enlargement. Since insufficient fetal mass can enter the birth canal to stimulate abdominal contractions, many breech presentations pass unrecognized for several hours, or even days, and when the problem is eventually recognized and corrected the calf is often stillborn.

Anasarca

Definition: extensive subcutaneous edema.

Clinical features: note the subcutaneous edema over the head, chest, and abdomen in the anasarca calf in 10.60. Although many cases can be delivered *per vaginum* by slow traction and generous lubrication, in this neglected case it led to maternal death from uterine rupture. Fetal anasarca in Ayrshires is hereditary. Other fetal monstrosities leading to dystocia include arthrogryposis (1.12), schistosomus reflexus (1.10), perosomus elumbus (absence of lumbar spine and pelvis), and ascites.

10.59. Dystocia: breech presentation with only tail visible

10.60. Anasarca with generalized edema of fetus

Uterine torsion

Clinical features: the anterior vagina can be seen to be rotated clockwise (10.61). About 75% of cases involve an anticlockwise torsion of 90–360°, detected clinically as a spiral effect on the vaginal wall. Torsion develops at the very end of pregnancy, during late first-stage or early second-stage labor, and is usually associated with a large calf. A live calf was delivered from this cow, following correction of the torsion, but many are stillborn.

Management: in most cases correction is by uterine manipulation *per vaginum*, or by rolling the cow in the same direction as the torsion. A proportion of cows also have incomplete cervical relaxation, resulting in dystocia, so that cesarian section may then prove the best option.

Postpartum complications

Normal, unassisted births result in few complications. However, after dystocia, particularly in cases of maternal disproportion involving considerable traction, complications are frequent. The most common is endometritis, which depresses subsequent fertility. Some of the more dramatic, but fortunately less frequent, complications illustrated here include vaginal wall rupture, uterine and

10.61. Uterine torsion with clockwise rotation of anterior vagina evident

10.62. Vaginal wall rupture and prolapse of perivaginal fat

10.64. Rectovaginal fistula with torn anal mucosa and vaginal wall

other prolapses, rectovaginal fistula, and septic vaginitis. A retained placenta can follow a normal parturition. Manual or endoscopic examination of discharges from the cervix and anterior vagina play an important role in prebreeding examination carried out as part of a herd fertility control program. A range of discharges encountered is illustrated with some gross uterine pathology.

Vaginal wall rupture and hemorrhage

Clinical features: vaginal wall rupture with hemorrhage is a common complication, seen especially in overfat heifers with large calves, insufficient lubrication during traction, and excessively rapid traction that does not permit normal vaginal and vulval dilation. Preventive episiotomy may be useful. Typically, the lateral vaginal wall tears approximately 10–20 cm from the vulval lips, dorsal to the external urethral orifice. A large mass of pelvic fat may prolapse through the tear and protrude through the vulval lips (10.62). Rupture of the vaginal artery, a branch of the internal pudendal artery that is easily palpated in the lateral vaginal wall at the point of tearing, can result in severe and often fatal hemorrhage within an hour of parturition (10.63). Fortunately, the blood vessel was identified and ligated in this heifer, although she subsequently developed a severe perivaginitis and localized pelvic peritonitis.

10.63. Hemorrhage from rupture of vaginal artery in heifer (Holstein)

Management: prevention is based on avoidance of dystocia (sire selection, dam nutrition) and careful delivery (ample lubricant, slow traction). The early recognition of the potential (episiotomy) or recent problem (vaginal tear, arterial rupture) may lead to corrective surgical steps. Delay, whether resulting from failure of observation or incorrect diagnosis, may result in death.

Rectovaginal fistula

Definition: traumatic connection between rectum and vagina.

Clinical features: rectovaginal fistula is a complication of dystocia, usually resulting from an oversized or malpresented fetus. In 10.64 (taken 5 days postpartum) the ventral anal mucosa is torn and there are extensive lacerations to the dorsal vaginal wall. The white material on the vaginal floor originates from intrauterine therapy. In the same cow 3 months later (10.65) the vaginal and anal lacerations had healed spontaneously, leaving a small, deformed area. Although fertility is usually reduced, due to development of pneumovagina or aspiration of feces into vagina, this cow became pregnant in each of the next 2 years. In an intraoperative view of another case (10.66), forceps opening the vulval lips display the extent of the tear between the rectum and vagina. The tissue has been cleaned and debrided in preparation for surgery.

Management: only small fistulae will heal spontaneously. Most require surgical repair. Large fistulae are untreatable. Remarkably, some untreated cows do remain fertile.

Septic vulvitis and vulvovaginitis

Clinical features: in 10.67 small, infected skin fissures are seen around the dorsal margin of the enlarged vulva, 4 days after the difficult delivery of an oversized calf. A length of placenta is seen in the ventral vulva. In severe cases of septic vulvitis the vulva is inflamed and

10

10.65. Healed rectovaginal fistula of cow of 10.64 after 3 months

10.67. Septic vulvitis and vulvovaginitis with infected skin fissures 4 days after dystocia

edematous, especially at the ventral commissure, and there is often a purulent hemorrhagic discharge from the vulva. A raised tail and tenesmus indicate discomfort. Although trauma at parturition is the commonest cause of vulval edema and cellulitis, the condition may also be the result of irritant feces caused by acute diarrhea.

Management: parenteral antibiotics, and also NSAIDs if pain and tenesmus are evident.

Retained placenta

Definition: expulsion of the placenta is the third stage of labor and normally occurs within 3–6 hours of fetal delivery. There is no precise time period for the definition of "retained placenta", but cases greater than 24 hours postpartum would qualify.

Clinical features: a retained placenta (10.68) is typically associated with factors that interfere with the third stage of labor, such as twins, prolonged parturition, excessive manual interference, abortion and premature calving, cows that are overfat or too thin, and vitamin, mineral and trace element deficiencies such as vitamin E and selenium. In recent years a new metabolic syndrome of high-yielding cows, associated with poor

10.66. Rectovaginal fistula prior to surgery (Italy)

10.68. Retained placenta 4 days postpartum

feed intakes postpartum, increased incidence of hypocalcemia, marked periparturient immunosuppression, and poor recovery from parturition has been recognized. It has produced a marked increase in placental retention, acute metritis, generalized toxemia, sickness, and deaths in postpartum animals.

In 10.68, taken 4 days postpartum, the placenta is turning pink due to autolysis, and the udder is stained with a foul uterine discharge.

Management: treatment is controversial! Attempt *gentle* traction after a few days, ensuring that maternal caruncles are not torn or damaged. Some consider that intrauterine antibiotics have no value, and may even be contraindicated because they delay normal placental dehiscence. Parenteral antibiotics and NSAIDs will assist resolution of any pyrexia and toxemia.

Prevention: attend to causative factors.

Vulval discharges, endometritis, metritis, and pyometra

Definition: endometritis involves an inflammation of the uterine lining. Metritis is a more generalized uterine inflammation often with secondary systemic pyrexia and toxemia. Pyometra is a closed purulent uterine inflammation with no vulval discharge.

Clinical features: vulval discharges may be associated with septic vulvovaginitis, a retained placenta, metritis, and endometritis. The type of discharge depends on the interval from calving to clinical examination, and on the degree of endometritis. Many discharges are normal and do not require treatment. Postestral blood in clear mucus is derived from uterine caruncle hemorrhage (10.69). A plug of cervical mucus (10.70), which may be seen immediately prepartum or postpartum, is normal. Discolored

10.70. Cervical mucus plug (normal)

mucus containing red-brown material (10.71) or globules of yellow detritus (10.72) are examples of lochia that would not normally be treated.

Endometritis is often first seen by the herdsman as a white, purulent vulval discharge from a cow lying in a cubicle, the material being deposited on the back of the standing (10.73). Clear mucus containing white flecks (10.74) is believed to indicate a low-grade endometritis.

10.69. Postestral blood in clear mucus (normal)

10.71. Vulval discharge of red-brown mucus

10.72. Vulval discharge of yellow detritus

10.73. Endometritis: purulent vulval discharge

A thick, white discharge typically indicates a significant endometritis, especially if accompanied by a foul smell. *Arcanobacterium pyogenes* and *Fusobacterium necrophorum* are commonly involved. Some cases have blood mixed with white globules (10.75).

10.74. Vulval discharge of clear mucus with white flecks

10.75. Endometritis: blood mixed with white globules of pus

10.76. Metritis: brown uterine discharge

Metritis is indicated by a stinking, brown discharge (10.76), particularly when its consistency is fluid and not mucoid. Affected animals often show systemic signs. For example, the cow in 10.77 was scouring and recumbent, with a sunken eye exposing congested conjunctiva. She died within a few hours as a result of toxemia and severe dehydration. On autopsy, the incised horn exposed necrotic cotyledons in brown, purulent fluid (10.78).

10.77. Sunken eye and congested conjunctiva in dying cow with severe metritis

10

10.78. Severe purulent endometritis and perimetritis in cow of 10.77

10.79. Vaginal prolapse: recent case

An area of caseopurulent perimetritis is seen above the incision, with discoloration and inflammation extending over the cervix and onto the pelvic vagina.

Management: vaginal examination and treatment of endometritis, where necessary, is an important part of routine herd fertility control, especially in dairy herds. Reference should be made to appropriate texts for details. Prevention depends on avoidance of dystocia, correct dam nutrition, especially in the periparturient period, control of metabolic disease, and proper hygiene at calving.

Prolapses of the female reproductive tract

Vaginal prolapse

Etiology: although it may occasionally be seen after parturition, vaginal prolapse typically occurs in older cows in late pregnancy. Caused by the pressure of abdominal contents forced into the pelvic cavity in late pregnancy, especially when the cow is in the lying position, vaginal prolapse is also associated with excess perivaginal fat, any type of vaginal or rectoanal irritation leading to tenesmus, older cows, estrogenic factors in feed leading to pelvic ligament relaxation, and with certain beef breeds, particularly Herefords.

Clinical features: the fresh, red appearance of the prolapse in 10.79 indicates that it is recent, with only mild congestion from exposure. A plug of cervical mucus is visible at the lower extremity. Prolonged cases become engorged and irritant, stimulating further straining. Prolapse of the vaginal wall with dystocia, as in 10.80, is uncommon. The vagina is the large everted structure protruding from the vulva and ending at the cervix (A). The dry fetus is still within the placenta, its forefoot being palpable through the partially dilated cervix.

Management: when the prolapse occurs only in the sitting or lying position it may be acceptable to do nothing, as it is likely to resolve following parturition. Permanent prolapses should be replaced under epidural analgesia and held in position with a deep transverse vulval suture to avoid swelling and irritation from external trauma. It is vital to check for the onset of parturition, when the suture should be released. In the case of 10.80 manual replacement and minimal assistance resulted in a normal birth. In herds with multiple cases the above predisposing factors should be examined carefully.

Cervical prolapse

Cervical prolapse is similar in etiology to vaginal prolapse. Small portions of the external os of the cervix may protrude through the vulva in cows in late pregnancy or early lactation (10.81), often disappearing when the animals stand up. A more advanced case is shown in the postpartum Shorthorn cow in 10.82. The external os is

10.80. Vaginal prolapse at dystocia with fetus in placenta

10

10.81. Partial cervical prolapse

edematous and grossly distended. A short length of vaginal wall is exposed between the cervix and vulva. Complete cervicovaginal prolapse may occur.

Management: small prolapses may resolve spontaneously. Larger masses should be cleansed, replaced, and held in place with transverse vulval sutures.

Uterine prolapse

Most cases of uterine prolapse occur within a few hours of calving. It is typically seen in older cows following

10.82. Cervical prolapse, severely edematous, and partial vaginal prolapse (Shorthorn)

10.83. Uterine prolapse of 2 hours' duration in young cow (Hereford)

dystocia or delivery of a large fetus, and may be associated with hypocalcemia or a retained placenta, but can also occur in heifers. The young Hereford cow in 10.83 has a prolapse of less than 2 hours' duration. The placenta is still attached and has a moist, fresh appearance. Most animals remain recumbent. Those which do move may traumatize the prolapse, increasing the risk of death from hemorrhage and shock. The Shorthorn cow in 10.84 has a complete prolapse of the uterus, vagina, and cervix. This is a rare condition and, like other cases involving the vagina and cervix, although the prolapse was replaced, she died within 12 hours as a result of shock and internal hemorrhage.

10.84. Prolapse of uterus, vagina, and cervix in cow (Shorthorn)

10

10.85. Pedunculated vaginal polyp

10.86. Aborted fetus at 7 months' gestation, unknown cause

Management: treat as emergency! The uterus can be protected from trauma and contamination by wrapping in a clean sheet, but many cows are best left lying undisturbed. Replace under epidural anesthesia with the recumbent cow in ventral recumbency with hind legs extended back, or by lifting hindquarters off the ground. Administer oxytocin, antibiotics, calcium borogluconate, and NSAIDs in possibly shocked cases. Most cows recover well, remain fertile, and recurrence at subsequent parturition is unlikely.

Vaginal and cervical polyps

Although not a postpartum complication, vaginal polyps are sometimes confused with an early prolapse. The vaginal polyp in 10.85 was pedunculated and protruded from the vulva in late pregnancy, disappearing postpartum when abdominal pressure was reduced.

Management: no treatment necessary.

Abortion and premature parturition

Definition: abortion has been defined as the premature expulsion of the products of conception, typically producing a dead calf. Premature calving occurs late in gestation, to give a live but weak calf, or a dead calf which would have been capable of an independent existence. Both phenomena may have similar infectious and noninfectious causes.

Clinical features: possible infectious factors include brucellosis, IBR, BVD, leptospirosis, vibriosis (*Campylobacter*), bluetongue, Schmallenberg virus (12.82) neosporosis, listeriosis, *Chlamydia*, *Coxiella*, aspergillosis, and, important in the Western USA, epizootic bovine abortion. Noninfectious factors include stress, lethal genes (e.g.,

arthrogryposis), poisons (e.g., locoweed (13.19) and mycotoxins), nutritional deficiencies (e.g., vitamin E, selenium, or iodine (2.51)), and physical injuries. The appearance of an aborted fetus (10.86 was aborted at 7 months of gestation) often gives little indication of the cause.

Many of the causes of abortion listed above are not illustrated, as they have no specific diagnostic features either in the placenta or fetus.

Differential diagnosis: specific diagnostic tests are necessary, but despite careful investigation, the cause of abortion is found in less than 25% of all cases.

Management: the dam occasionally needs treatment for endometritis (p. 194). Identify the cause. Vaccines are available against BVD, IBR, and leptospirosis. Control possible oral ingestion of *Aspergillus*, *Listeria*, and toxins. Consider culling carrier cows with *Neospora*.

Premature calf

In addition to a reduced body size, the premature (7 months) Simmental crossbred calf in 10.87 shows hyperemia (reddening) of the mouth and nostrils, soft hooves, and a short, "staring" coat. Most causes of

10.87. Premature (7 months' gestation) calf with mucosal hyperemia and short coat (Simmental cross)

10

10.88. Mummified fetus, 4 months' gestation

10.89. Brucellosis: thickened placenta with white necrotic foci on cotyledons

abortion mentioned previously can also produce premature births. Leptospirosis was the most probable cause in this case as the dam had a titer of 1:1600 to *Leptospira hardjo*.

Mummified fetus

The fetus in 10.88 died at approximately 4 months of gestation, but was not expelled until 8 months. Note the sunken eye sockets and the characteristic dry, chocolate-brown color of the decomposing fetus and placenta. BVD and *Neospora* are two common causes of mummification. Stress in early pregnancy may predispose. Certain bulls, especially Jerseys, may genetically produce an increased incidence of mummified fetuses.

Brucellosis (contagious abortion, Bang's disease)

Definition: brucellosis is a bacterial infection caused in cattle by *Brucella abortus*.

Clinical features: susceptible cattle ingest material from an infected fetus, placenta, or uterine discharge and typically abort between 7 and 8 months of gestation. A marked placentitis may occur in the form of small, white, necrotic foci on the cotyledons and thickening of the intercotyledonary placenta (10.89). Organisms are shed in milk as well as uterine discharges. Most cows only abort once, although they may remain persistent carriers and excrete *Brucella* at subsequent normal parturitions. Retained placenta, endometritis, and infertility are common complications.

In the bull, the testicles (10.33) and seminal vesicles may be affected, although infection is only rarely present in the semen. Brucellosis is transmissible to humans, and is a notifiable disease in many countries.

Differential diagnosis: other causes of abortion, e.g., trichomoniasis, leptospirosis, IBR, neosporosis. Diagnosis by blood agglutination tests, milk ring test, CF tests.

Management: many countries have national eradication programs involving testing, elimination of reactors, and calfhood vaccination.

Mycotic abortion

Definition: systemic mycoses (aspergillosis, rarely candidiasis and zygomycosis) tend to be sporadic nonspecific syndromes which can lead to abortion.

Clinical features: moldy silage which was accidentally fed to 20 cows in late pregnancy led to systemic aspergillosis. Hematogenous spread, leading to fetal infection, produced 3 abortions in 10 days. *Aspergillus* was isolated from the fetuses. In some cases, small, circular, ringworm-like lesions (10.90) are seen on the fetal skin. There may also be a pronounced thickening of the placenta and necrosis of the cotyledons (10.91). Abortions tend to occur from 4 months to term, and in some countries are more common in the winter months. *Mucor* species may also be involved, producing a yellow

10.90. Mycotic abortion: *Aspergillus* isolated from "ringworm-like" skin lesions

10.91. Mycotic abortion: thickened placenta and necrosis of cotyledon

10.92. Mycotic abortion: yellow placental discoloration due to *Mucor* spp.

discoloration and degeneration of the serosal surface of the placenta (10.92).

Diagnosis: based on skin lesions, demonstrations of hyphae in fetal dermatitis, especially on eyelids, placental lesions, bronchopneumonia, and possibly abomasal contents. There may be no specific lesions if the abortion has been caused by ingestion of mycotoxin and not by a primary mycotic infection. Diagnosis is then based on the history of exposure, possible concurrent presence of other clinical signs (abdominal pain, digestive upsets, lower limb swelling), and demonstration of mycotoxin in the feed.

Management: improve feed preservation and storage to reduce ingestion of moldy feed.

10

Udder and teat disorders

Introduction

The dairy cow is bred and fed to produce large volumes of milk. With the metabolic stress of high performance and the physical effects of being milked and handled two or three times daily, it is not surprising that the udder and teats are subject to a wide variety of disorders. The primary disease, mastitis, is of worldwide economic importance and much money is spent on its prevention, treatment and control. The first part of the chapter deals with mastitis in lactating and dry cows, and describes changes that may be seen in milk. The second part illustrates teat lesions, including a wide variety of viral infections, notably bovine herpes mammillitis, cowpox and pseudocowpox, vesicular stomatitis, and fibropapillomas (warts). Other systemic diseases that also affect the teats, e.g., foot-and-mouth disease, are covered elsewhere (p. 221).

Because of their anatomical position, especially in cows with pendulous udders, teats are vulnerable to injuries, eczema, and other physical influences. These problems are considered in the third part of this chapter, although changes associated with photosensitization are covered elsewhere (3.5). The final part of the chapter includes miscellaneous conditions of the udder.

Congenital conditions

Supernumerary teats

Clinical features: supernumerary teats are a congenital condition. They may be found between the front and rear teats, and/or attached to the udder behind the rear teats (11.1), or to the base or side of one of the main teats, where they can interfere with milking. They are typically, shorter than normal teats, and have thinner walls. They may connect to the sinus of an existing teat, or, more commonly, have a separate supernumerary gland.

Management: as such teats are unsightly, may interfere with milking, and can develop mastitis, they are normally removed with curved scissors early in life. Care is necessary to identify the correct teat.

Blind quarters

Definition: a quarter that produces no milk.

Clinical features: blind quarters in heifers with non-patent teats can be either congenital or acquired. There are two congenital forms, one in which there is a total absence of the teat canal, but the teat fills with milk, and less

11.1. Two supernumerary teats behind rear teats

commonly a second where there is a persistent membrane between the teat cistern and canal at the teat base, and no milk can be palpated in the teat. The acquired form, when a thickened central core is palpable in the teat canal, may be caused by undetected summer mastitis (11.2) or trauma from being suckled as a calf (2.14). The associated quarter may be swollen immediately postpartum due to accumulated milk, but this later regresses to be smaller than the other quarters. In mature cows a blind quarter may occasionally arise from chronic mastitis in the previous lactation, although in many animals a prolonged dry period often results in self-cure. Visible unevenness of quarters occurs in around 60% of milking animals, varying with age, stage of lactation, and mastitis history.

Mastitis

Summer mastitis

Definition: this form of mastitis, typically seen in non-lactating cows and heifers, invariably leads to extensive parenchymal damage and loss of the quarter. An infectious condition commonly involving *Arcanobacterium pyogenes* and many other possible organisms, it is transmitted by the sheep head fly, *Hydrotaea irritans*. Some cases may occur in lactating cows secondary to teat sphincter trauma.

Clinical features: this endemic form of suppurative mastitis, with a characteristic foul odor, typically occurs sporadically in mid–late summer in Europe, because the vector *H. irritans* is active during July–September. Mild cases become only slightly ill, whilst the more severely affected cows are dull, pyrexic, and anorexic. They may abort, or produce weakly calves at term. Acute, untreated cases may die. Very few quarters recover, although cases are very occasionally mild enough to pass unrecognized until calving, when the affected quarter is non-functional ("blind") and the teat is palpably thickened. Occasionally summer mastitis is seen in a bull or a young calf.

The Charolais heifer in 11.2 is an early case, showing distension of the left hind quarter, which was typically hard and sore, with a prominent, turgid teat. In more advanced cases, the infection may burst through the udder, as shown in the right hind quarter in 11.3. A thickening of the central teat canal was palpable, the quarter was very hard, and yellow pus with a pungent odor was discharging from the teat and udder.

Management: parenteral treatment with antibiotics possibly and NSAIDs will reduce the systemic effects. Local antibiotic treatment of the quarter is rarely successful, but frequent stripping or surgical drainage using a longitudinal teat incision may prevent udder abscessation.

Control: dry cow therapy with longacting intramammary antibiotics, internal teat sealants, fly repellents, and keeping cattle away from known fly areas, or housing them during the period of risk. In high-risk areas fly repellents should ideally be applied to the udder weekly.

11

11.2 Summer mastitis: left hind quarter and teat thickened in heifer (Charolais)

11.3. Sumer mastitis: suppurative mastitis in dry cow has burst through skin

Acute mastitis

Peracute and acute mastitis are most commonly seen in the first few weeks after calving and are often the result of periparturient immune suppression. Disease may result from recrudescence of dormant dry period infections, or from new intramammary infections during lactation. Cases can occur throughout lactation at a lower frequency. In most cases peracute mastitis with toxemia results from coliform infections. Similarly, in acute mastitis, environmental organisms such as coliforms (e.g., *Escherichia coli*) or *Streptococcus uberis* are frequently involved. Immune suppression occasionally leads to acute disease from "contagious" mastitis organisms such as staphylococci, which are carried on the skin or in the udder of affected cows and transmitted to other cows during milking.

Clinical features: the most prominent sign of acute mastitis is an enlarged, hard, hot and painful quarter, which may be apparent before any changes are visible in the milk. In some cases, a brown serous discharge may be seen on the surface of the affected quarter and teat, as in the lactating Friesian cow in 11.4. A section of an affected udder (11.5), shows deep red inflammation of the teat cistern and teat canal mucosa. There is prominent subcutaneous edema and the skin at the tip of the teat is congested. Changes of this nature can lead to gangrene. The yellow foci (A) in the udder parenchyma are pockets of pus. In 11.6 the teat of the affected quarter is swollen with areas of hemorrhage. There is an obvious area of gangrene affecting the udder skin, which is dry, cracked, and cold. This cow was severely ill with an eventually fatal toxemia, although in less extensive cases the necrotic portion of the udder will slough and recovery is still possible. Such cases should not be confused with udder bruising (11.7).

Advanced gangrene (11.8) leads to cold, damp teat skin. Although mastitis was limited to the left forequarter

11.5. Acute mastitis: inflammatory changes in teat cistern and mucosa, severe skin edema

11.6. Acute mastitis, early gangrenous changes

11.4. Acute mastitis: enlarged quarter with serous discharge on skin

11.7. Bruising of udder with skin discoloration and enlarged forequarter

11

11.8. Advanced gangrene of udder: peracute case with slough of skin around affected quarter (A)

11.10. Chronic mastitis: large nodules are chronic staphylococcal abscesses within mammary parenchyma

(A), the entire udder was blue, edematous, and cold to the touch. Adjacent to the affected teat is a skin slough and red exudate. The secretion from the udder was a deep port-wine color and was mixed with gas. The cow had been normal when milked 12 hours previously, indicating the peracute onset of disease. In cases of nonfatal, gangrenous mastitis the overlying skin (11.9), or even the entire affected quarter, sloughs slowly in 1–2 months.

Management: intramammary antibiotics, combined with parenteral antibiotics, fluid therapy and NSAIDs for more acute cases. Continual stripping of affected quarters, and parenteral oxytocin allegedly improves recovery rate. Prevention depends on reducing pathogen concentration at the teat orifice and correct machine function. Environmental hygiene, correct premilking teat preparation, avoidance of mechanical trauma to the teat sphincter (11.32, 11.33), and minimization of teat end impacts are all important points. Standard texts give details.

Chronic mastitis

Definition: *Streptococcus agalactiae*, *S. dysgalactiae*, *S. uberis*, staphylococci, *Mycoplasma*, *Arcanobacterium pyogenes*, and other bacteria can produce a chronic mastitis, manifested as "clots" in the milk (11.14), with or without palpable udder changes.

Clinical features: the Friesian cow in 11.10 has large, hard nodules protruding from the udder, with two in the right quarter and one in the left. These are chronic, intramammary, staphylococcal abscesses. Staphylococci were cultured from the milk, which had a high cell count and gave a strongly positive reaction to the California mastitis test. Such advanced cases, which are usually unresponsive to treatment, are dangerous carriers and should be culled. If only one quarter is affected, that quarter may be dried off otherwise infection will be transferred to other quarters and other cows at milking. The Friesian cow in 11.11 had a blind quarter, having had mastitis in the previous lactation. The front left teat is slightly smaller than the others, and the associated quarter has totally atrophied.

Management: treatment options are as for environmental infections. Control of contagious mastitis rests on reducing cow-to-cow spread of infection during the

11

11.9. Gangrenous mastitis: nonfatal case with massive skin slough

11.11 "Blind" quarter: front left teat and quarter atrophied

11.12. Blood in milk: newly calved cow with isolated clots

milking process. Milking hygiene (gloves, liners, paper towels, etc.), early detection and treatment of cases, thorough postmilking teat disinfection, correct milking machine function, dry cow antibiotic therapy, and culling are important control measures. Raised cell counts in the bulk tank milk may lead to financial penalties.

Mastitic changes in milk

Milk is thicker and more viscous during the dry period and immediately postpartum (i.e., colostrum). Its character also changes in mastitis. Although specific types of mastitic infection frequently lead to similar changes in milk, the appearance of the milk is not pathognomonic, and bacteriological examination is required to confirm the causative organism and to determine the antibiotic sensitivity.

Blood in milk

Clinical features: true blood clots are the characteristic feature of blood in milk. They may be present in slightly pink-tinged milk (11.12) or, in more severe cases, in a secretion that is almost totally red (11.13). Seen only in newly calved cows, or after trauma, the condition

11.14. Mastitic milk: watery milk with occasional clots

usually resolves spontaneously. Herd outbreaks of unknown etiology may occur.

Management: no treatment has been found to be consistently useful. Incomplete milking leading to increased intramammary pressure is believed to assist in hemostasis, but as this increases the risk of a new quarter infection, prophylactic antibiotic cover should be given.

Mastitic milk

Clinical features: watery, translucent milk with occasional clots (11.14) is typical of a mild mastitis such as that caused by *S. agalactiae* or *S. dysgalactiae*. Normal milk may be totally absent in severe staphylococcal (11.15) or *Arcanobacterium pyogenes* infections, when the secretion consists of thick clots suspended in a clear, serous fluid. Summer mastitis (often *A. pyogenes*) invariably produces a thick secretion with a characteristic pungent odor.

A light brown, serum-colored secretion is typical of *Escherichia coli* infection (11.16), while acute gangrenous mastitis (e.g., acute staphylococcal) may produce a red or brown homogenous secretion (11.17), often mixed with gas.

11

11.13. Blood in milk: severe case

11.15. Mastitic milk: thick clots in clear serous fluid

11.16. Mastitic milk: brownish fluid typical of coliform infection

11.17. Mastitic milk: red or brown homogenous fluid with gas typical of acute gangrenous mastitis

Infectious teat conditions

Teats are affected by two pox viruses: pseudocowpox (paravaccinia), a mild infection that occurs throughout the world, and cowpox (vaccinia), which is now extremely rare. Both are transmissible to humans. The parapoxvirus of pseudocowpox is related to bovine papular stomatitis

(4.13, 4.14). Bovine herpes mammillitis (BHM) is a much more severe infection and may be confused clinically with the teat changes associated with necrotic dermatitis (udder seborrhea). Other viral infections producing teat lesions include vesicular stomatitis (11.26, 11.27), fibro-papillomas (11.29–11.31), bluetongue (12.19), foot-and-mouth disease (12.2), and rinderpest (12.9). Teats are also subject to physical injury, chapping, and eczema, often exacerbated by cold, wet conditions and poor milking machine function. Examples include hyperkera-tosis and "black spot" of the teat sphincter (11.40), summer (licking) sores (11.42), trauma, and photosensi-tization (3.5).

Bovine herpes mammillitis (BHM)

Definition: infectious ulcerative dermatitis of teats and udder skin caused by bovine herpesvirus-2.

Clinical features: BHM initially produces fluid-filled vesicles, seen in the center and toward the tip of the teat in 11.18. The overlying epithelium is tense and white. The initial vesicles easily rupture to expose raw, ulcerated areas (seen between the two vesicles in 11.18), which coalesce and later become covered by thick scabs (11.19). The condition is so painful that it is often impossible to milk affected cows (compare pseudocowpox, 11.20–11.24). BHM tends to occur in outbreaks, most commonly in first-calving heifers soon after calving, and secondary mastitis is a major problem. Calves sucking affected cows can develop ulcers on the muzzle, buccal mucosa, and tongue, and may become febrile and lose weight. Many cases occur in the first few weeks postpartum and are thought to result from immune suppression in the periparturient carrier cow. Persistent herd infection is possible. Lifelong immunity follows recovery.

Differential diagnosis: necrotic dermatitis (11.53), bluetongue (12.19), FMD (12.6), pseudocowpox (11.20).

Management: iodophor teat disinfectants may help to prevent spread. Isolation of affected cows has not been useful.

11.18. Bovine herpes mammillitis (BHM): teat with typical vesicles, unruptured and ruptured

11.19. Bovine herpes mammillitis: later stage with scabs on teats

11.20. Pseudocowpox (parapox): small, painless papule on teat

11.21. Pseudocowpox: characteristic circular or horseshoe-shaped areas and marginal scab formation

Pseudocowpox (parapox)

Definition: teat infection caused by a paravaccinia virus.

Clinical features: pseudocowpox is a worldwide infection, spreading slowly within a herd. Both the teats (primarily) and the udder may be affected, and "milker's nodules" may occur on the fingers of humans. An individual cow may remain clinically affected for several months and, as immunity is short-lived, repeated attacks can occur every 2–3 years.

The disease starts as a small, painless papule affecting the superficial layers of the skin (11.20). After 7–10 days the lesion enlarges from the periphery to produce characteristic circular or horseshoe-shaped areas, delineated by small, red scabs (11.21). The affected area feels rough, but is not painful, and milking is not usually impeded. Scabs slowly resolve in the healing phase (11.22), although in some cases (11.23) nodules may develop. In rare cases the lesion develops a very rough, slightly moist, papilliform appearance, with several elevated and confluent masses (11.24).

Differential diagnosis: bluetongue (12.19), cowpox (11.25), vesicular stomatitis (11.26, 11.27), bovine herpes mammillitis (11.18, 11.19).

Management: milking hygiene, use of good-quality teat dips with emollients, and reduction of teat skin trauma help to prevent the spread of infection.

Cowpox (bovine orthopox)

Definition: benign contagious teat infection caused by an Orthopoxvirus closely related to smallpox in humans.

Clinical features: cowpox produces painful vesicles on the skin of the teats and the udder. 11.25 illustrates three teat skin vesicles which have ruptured, exposing the underlying granulation tissue. As with the two previous conditions spread is by teat cups and milkers' hands. Cowpox is now extremely rare and the infection is limited to Western Europe.

Differential diagnosis: pseudocowpox (11.20–11.24), BHM (11.18, 11.19), vesicular stomatitis (11.26, 11.27), necrotic dermatitis.

Management: general measures as for BHM.

11.22. Pseudocowpox: healing scabs

11.23. Teat nodules in pseudocowpox

Vesicular stomatitis

Definition: infectious viral (rhabdovirus) disease causing stomatitis (4.11), sometimes with lesions on the udder, teats, coronary band, and interdigital space.

Clinical features: vesicular stomatitis is found only in North and South America, and is transmitted by mosquitoes and biting flies. The reservoir hosts are American forest ground mammals. Excessive salivation is frequently the first sign. It primarily produces mouth lesions (4.11), but lesions can also occur on the teats. Multiple, irregular-shaped, white vesicles, some of which have ruptured, cover much of the teat skin in 11.26

11.25. Cowpox (bovine orthopox): granulation tissue following ruptured teat vesicles

and 11.27. Uncomplicated cases heal within 2 weeks. Recovered animals are immune for 12–18 months.

Differential diagnosis: foot-and-mouth disease (12.2– 12.7), bovine papular stomatitis (4.13, 4.14). Diagnosis is usually by ELISA and CF tests.

Management: disease should be notified to national animal health authorities. Symptomatic treatment and restriction on animal movement are usual.

11.24. Pseudocowpox: uncommon rough, moist, proliferative masses

11.26. Vesicular stomatitis: irregular vesicles, some ruptured on teats

11.27. Vesicular stomatitis: ruptured teat end vesicles and granulation tissue

Foot-and-mouth disease

Clinical features: though not a primary clinical sign, cows with FMD in the acute phase may develop multiple vesicles on the teats, in some cases becoming almost impossible to milk. 11.28 shows multiple teat vesicles in a Kuwait cow (see also p. 221).

Fibropapillomas (warts)

Clinical features: caused by different strains of papoviruses, warts are common among groups of pregnant and first-lactation heifers, typically over the lower part of the teat. Some have a "feathery," keratinized, and papilliform appearance (11.29) and can be easily pulled off. Others are more nodular (11.30) and tightly adherent to the skin. Mixed infections may occur (11.31). Fibropapillomas close to the teat orifice and sphincter (11.31)

11.29. Fibropapillomas (warts): feathery and papilliform types

11.30. Fibropapilloma: nodular type on teat

11.28. Foot-and-mouth disease: multiple teat vesicles (Kuwait)

11.31. Fibropapilloma: mixed papilliform and nodular teat lesions

11

interfere with milking and predispose animals to teat stenosis and mastitis. In some animals the condition is so extensive that the animals are impossible to milk. Flies are considered to be important vectors for transmission. Warts can also occur on the skin (3.44), eye (8.43), and penis (10.19).

Management: "feathery warts" and those with a distinct stalk can be pulled off surprisingly easily and produce minimal hemorrhage. No vaccines are very effective though autogenous products seem better than commercial vaccines. Many warts slowly resolve in the first lactation.

Noninfectious teat conditions

The teats are susceptible to trauma from machine milking, the environment, and physical and chemical factors. Any damage is of considerable economic importance as it predisposes to mastitis.

Teat end callosity (hyperkeratosis, canal eversion)

Clinical features: in the normal bovine teat, the canal sphincter and orifice should show minimal protrusion from the teat end. Teat end callosity and subsequent hyperkeratosis, i.e., protrusion of keratin fronds or filaments, is always the result of faulty machine milking. Hyperkeratosis is more common in pointed than in cylindrical-shaped teats, in higher-yielding cows, and in early to mid lactation, and although many teats resolve over the dry period, repeated trauma from one lactation to the next has a cumulative effect. In 11.32 the teat canal is seen as a raised, pale, bulbous swelling of the circular sphincter area, with small, protruding fragments of dry, keratinized material. This indicates a grade 2 hyperkeratosis (grades 0–5 indicate normal to severe change; other scoring systems are also used, e.g., smooth ring (SR), rough ring (RR), and very rough ring (VR)). 11.33 shows a grade 3 callosity, with keratin fronding around the entire everted teat canal circumference. Milking machine trauma also produced the dry, circular, hemorrhagic areas seen at the teat apex. Affected teats are often hard and

11.33. Teat end callosity: extensive frond formation, grade 3

edematous, a further effect of machine-induced trauma. Advanced cases, which predispose to new intramammary infections in both the dry period and in lactation, show severe keratinization (11.34, grade 5), which may precede black spot.

Management: where multiple teats in a significant proportion of the herd (e.g., mean teat score greater than 1.0, or more than 20% rough and very rough rings, and more than 10% very rough rings) are involved, teat end callosity/hyperkeratosis will invariably be caused by defective machine milking, e.g., a fault either in the way in which the plant is set up (including excess vacuum, inadequate "d" phase pulsation, and poor cluster removal), or the way in which it is used (including prolonged "unit on" times and poor udder preparation leading to delayed let-down). Healing takes place after correction of the fault(s), which must therefore be identified and urgently corrected.

Teat base compression rings

Definition: a compression ring at the base of the liner caused by excess liner pressure

Clinical features: all four teats (11.35) on this freshly calved heifer are swollen and edematous. They will be palpably hard. Longitudinal scratch marks on the medial

11.32. Teat end callosity (teat canal eversion) with dry keratinized protrusions, grade 2

11.34. Teat end callosity: severe keratinization, grade 5

11.35. Bruising rings from teat base compression

11.37. Hemorrhage, teat apex compression

aspect of the right fore teat are calf teeth marks from suckling. There is a circumferential ring around the base of the left hind teat, at the teat-udder junction. This constriction of the teat can reduce milk flow rates, increase "unit on" time, and indirectly lead to teat end damage.

Management: a small compression ring in a freshly calved heifer may be acceptable, especially if the udder is edematous. If present on a herd basis, predisposing causes (including ill-fitting liners (inflations), excess plant vacuum, lightweight claws leading to liner "creep", and excess udder edema) should be investigated and controlled.

Apex compression and teat end slough

Clinical features: much less common than teat end callosity, this condition (11.36) is also caused by machine milking trauma. Initial changes of hyperemia and thickening (right teat of 11.36) of the teat skin may progress to marked hemorrhage at the teat end (11.37), ischemic necrosis, and a superficial slough over the teat canal, extending 10–15 mm dorsally (11.36, left). Only superficial skin layers slough, and although the circumferential slough is remarkably symmetrical, healing is quite rapid once the milking machine trauma has been removed, leaving an obvious skin change similar to a

burn. The risk of new intramammary infections and mastitis is high.

Chaps and fissures

Clinical features: "teat chaps" are skin (epidermal) fissures. They may result from repeated exposure to wet, cold winds, inappropriate postmilking teat disinfectants, teeth damage caused by a suckling calf, or irritant chemicals. Chaps, as in 11.38, may affect the whole of the teat, and when skin defenses are compromised in this way, mastitis organisms such as *Staphylococcus aureus* and *Streptococcus dysgalactiae* may proliferate. A degree of compression at the teat end, seen at cluster removal, is a normal feature of machine milking. In advanced cases skin fissures or "chaps" develop at the teat orifice (11.39).

11.36. Teat end slough: hyperemic thickened teat (right), superficial teat slough (left)

11.38. Teat "chaps:" multiple parallel skin fissures

11

11.39.   Skin fissures or "chaps" from over-worn liners

These may be caused by liners (inflations) that are too narrow or too short for the average teat length, poor pulsation, excess plant vacuum, or possibly excessively worn liners (inflations) producing a "slapping" effect on the teat end during pulsation, as the liner always opens and closes in the same horizontal plane.

Black spot

Definition: black spot describes a proliferative necrotic dermatitis of the teat end around the sphincter.

Clinical features: black necrotic tissue is clearly visible extending to the left in 11.40. The lesion often

11.40.   "Black spot" with adjacent skin fissure or teat "chap"

11.41.   Teat trauma with ulceration near orifice and "black spot"

follows environmental trauma (e.g., overmilking, excessive vacuum fluctuation, wet teats exposed to a chilling wind), leading to damage of the teat orifice, which is then secondarily infected with *Staphylococcus aureus* or *Fusobacterium necrophorum* (see also 11.41). The skin fissure adjacent to the black spot lesion in 11.40 is a teat chap. A more typical case, with a moist, wet, inflamed area surrounding the teat canal, is shown in 11.41.

Management: on a herd basis, identify and correct predisposing causes. Treatment of individual cases with debriding agents, antiseptic creams, and emollients may help, or dry off the quarter to prevent further machine-induced trauma. Either course of action carries a high mastitis risk.

Summer sores and teat eczema

Clinical features: summer sores are eczematous lesions that result from excessive licking, and may be secondary to irritation caused by flies. First seen as irregular-shaped areas of moist, wet eczema at the teat base, they may spread to involve almost the entire teat (11.42), when they can be very painful. 11.42 shows islets of residual epithelium in the granulation tissue, especially toward the tip of the teat, and a serous exudate. Simple sunburn producing a thickening of teat skin may also occur (3.4).

Differential diagnosis: differentiation from bovine herpes mammillitis (11.19), chemical damage (11.47), sunburn, fire burn (3.75), and necrotic dermatitis (11.51) is difficult at the stage seen in 11.42.

Management: fly preventive measures, emollients.

Ischemic teat necrosis

Definition: a superficial inflammation of the teat skin, which, in advanced cases, causes intense irritation.

Clinical features: the initial lesion is seen as a dark area of dry dermatitis invariably medially at the base of

11.42. Teat eczema or summer sores involving almost entire teat

the teat (11.43, in this case the left hind). The lesion expands from the periphery and may cover the whole of the medial aspect of the teat. Advanced cases (11.44) become intensely irritant, and the teat is licked excessively, often such that the whole teat is removed by self-inflicted injury. In 11.44 the right fore teat appears normal but the left fore is swollen and hemorrhagic. Note the licked hair on the adjacent abdominal wall. Much of the right hind teat has been removed by licking, and the left hind teat is totally absent. There is extensive blood staining on the medial metatarsal region below the hock.

Differential diagnosis: the initial dry eczema is almost pathognomonic although later cases may be indistinguishable from summer sores (11.42) and their differentials including bovine herpes mammillitis (11.18, 11.19), chemical damage (11.47), sunburn, and fire burn (3.75).

Management: the cause is currently unknown. Early cases are treated symptomatically by topical steroids and emollients, ensuring that the milking cluster is on for a minimal period. NSAIDs can be used if the acute syndrome starts, but there seems to be little that prevents total teat removal.

Physical teat trauma

Clinical features: because of their position, teats are very prone to injury, especially in cows with turgid or pendulous udders. Barbed wire often produces multiple lacerations and may leave a horizontal flap of skin (11.45). This flap tends to be pulled downward when the teat cups are removed at milking, thus retarding healing. Amputation of the skin flap promotes healing. Superficial epidermal abrasions (11.46) cause few problems, although this teat had been injured in a previous lactation, leaving a fistula (A) of the cistern at its base. Trauma can cause complete loss of a large area of teat skin, which often heals surprisingly well. Injuries involving the teat sphincter carry a high risk of both mastitis and stenosis of the orifice.

11.43. Ischemic teat necrosis—mild

11.44. Ischemic teat necrosis—severe

11.45. Teat trauma from barbed wire injury, leaving skin flap

11

11.46. Teat fistula (A) of milk cistern and recent trauma

Chemical teat trauma

Clinical features: the degree of damage depends partly on the chemical involved. Common causes are acids (e.g., formic acid used as a cluster flush, lactic acid from teat dips, and phosphoric acid from bulk tank cleaner and milk stone remover) and alkalis (e.g., sodium hydroxide and other plant-cleaning chemicals, hydrated lime and power station ash used as free stall bedding). These are either mistakenly applied to teats as a postmilking disinfectant or teat contact is made when lying. Note the raw, open sores on the left hind teat of 11.47, and scab formation at both the base and especially the apex of the right teat where it predisposes to mastitis. This damage was caused by accidental use of concentrated lactic acid as a dip.

11.47. Chemical damage to teat

11.48. Teat cistern granuloma ("pea") being manually expressed through teat orifice

Management: identify and remove the chemical causing the burn. Individual cows need a high-emollient dip and minimal "unit on" time.

Teat cistern granuloma (pea)

Definition: discrete fibrogranulomatous mass which may float free in teat cistern or be attached to the endothelium.

Clinical features: free-floating, irregular, rubbery masses of fibrocollagenous material ("peas") may develop in the teat cistern and pass down to the sphincter, thus obstructing the milk flow. As in 11.48, some can be manually expressed from a surgically dilated teat orifice. Others remain attached to the teat mucosa, cannot be so easily removed, and may continue to block the teat canal. A variety of shapes, sizes, and colors is found (11.49). All have a rubbery texture, measure about 5–10 mm long, and, as many are red, they probably originate from blood clots.

Conditions of the udder skin and subcutis

Udder impetigo (udder acne)

Definition: a staphylococcal dermatitis of the teats and udder skin.

11.49. Three teat granulomata ("peas") about 5–10 mm long

11

11.50. Udder impetigo ("udder acne") with multiple red papules

Clinical features: small, red papules are seen on the udder of the Friesian in 11.50. They sometimes coalesce to produce an exudative dermatitis that can spread onto the teats and may develop a foul odor. A coagulase-positive *Staphylococcus* was isolated in this case.

Differential diagnosis (of advanced teat cases): bovine herpes mammillitis (11.18), necrotic dermatitis (11.51).

Management: topical antibiotic therapy is surprisingly effective.

Necrotic dermatitis (udder seborrhea)

Clinical features: this dermatitis occurs in the first 1–2 weeks after calving, especially in heifers, and is associated with excessive prepartum udder edema, leading to

11.52. Necrotic dermatitis with red-brown ischemic udder skin and dirty serous discharge (caudal view)

skin ischemia and necrosis. Mild cases (11.51) develop a moist and often foul-smelling superficial dermatitis laterally in the contact area between the udder and thigh. In more advanced cases (11.52) the ischemic udder skin turns reddish-purple and produces a dirty, serous exudate, similar to some cases of acute or peracute mastitis (11.4). A dry, scaly dermatitis (11.53) with extensive thickening of the teats may make some animals impossible to milk. Note the residual cutaneous edema cranial to the udder in this heifer.

Differential diagnosis: severe udder impetigo (staphylococcal dermatitis) (11.50), bluetongue (12.19), bovine herpes mammillitis (11.18).

Management: cleanse lesions, removing debris, and apply topical antibiotics or antiseptics.

Prevention: careful transition feed management, avoid overfat cows, and increase exercise to reduce mammary edema.

11

11.51. Necrotic dermatitis or intertrigo: mild, moist, superficial dermatitis

11.53. Necrotic dermatitis: dry, scaly dermatitis with teat thickening

11.54. Necrotic dermatitis: intertrigo between udder and ventral body wall, with deep exudative changes

11.55. Ventral abdominal edema in postparturient heifer (Holstein)

Ulcerative mammary dermatitis (UMD, intertrigo)

Definition: a moist dermatitis in the skin between the two forequarters and the ventral body wall.

Clinical features: also called intertrigo, the lesion is a deep, moist, and exudative dermatitis with a pungent odor (11.54). Necrotic debris is seen in the center. Organisms closely resembling the spirochetes of digital dermatitis have been identified in some cases.

Management: thoroughly clean the lesion and apply topical antibiotics or antiseptics. Some persist for several weeks or months.

Udder bruising

Definition: subcutaneous hemorrhage in the udder, usually in the ventral areas, associated with trauma.

Clinical features: in 11.7 the forequarter is obviously enlarged, the front teat deviates medially, and a blue discoloration is seen on the lower half of both quarters. The cow was, however, bright and alert, there were no visible changes in the milk, and the skin remained warm. Such cases should not be confused with gangrenous mastitis (11.6).

Udder and ventral abdominal edema

Clinical features: a physiological periparturient condition, extensive subcutaneous edema is seen cranial to the udder of the Holstein heifer in 11.55, 2 days after calving. In advanced cases it may extend to the sternum. Typically, edema is demonstrated as "pitting" when pressure is applied. Digital pressure on the rear of an edematous udder (11.56) creates a depression (seen to the left of the finger (A)) which persists for 30–60 seconds after the finger has been withdrawn.

Differential diagnosis: abscess, hematoma.

Management: overfeeding, excessive salt and other mineral intakes, an overfat prepartum condition, heredity, and lack of exercise are among the factors contributing to excess edema and require appropriate measures. A sudden onset of edema in one or more quarters in mid lactation cows, with unknown etiology, has recently been reported.

Rupture of udder ligaments (dropped udder)

The suspensory apparatus of the udder consists of superficial and deep lateral ligaments, an anterior ligament and a fibroelastic median ligament. Any can stretch or rupture.

Clinical features: rupture of the median and lateral suspensory apparatus. The 6-year-old Guernsey cow in 11.57 had calved 4 weeks previously, and had suddenly developed a grossly pendulous udder as a result of sudden rupture of both the lateral and median suspensory apparatus (ligaments) of the udder. Note that the ventral udder surface is considerably below the level of

11.56. "Pitting" edema demonstrated on udder (USA)

11.57. Rupture of udder ligaments (dropped udder) in cow, 4 weeks postpartum (Guernsey, 6 years old)

11.58. Rupture of anterior ligament of udder

the hock. The outward direction of the teats is a mechanical result of the loss of the median ligamentous support of the udder. There was no evidence of mastitis. Autopsy examination revealed a massive hematoma surrounding the ligamentous rupture between the ventral body wall and the gland parenchyma.

Rupture of the anterior ligament is seen in the freshly calved Friesian cow (11.58) which suddenly developed this massive midline swelling cranial to the udder, filling the normal space between the forequarters and ventral body wall. Note that the front teats are so splayed that milking is impossible. The milk vein (A) runs along the top of the picture, and may occasionally rupture internally, leading to quite severe anemia.

Differential diagnosis: acute mastitis, ventral abdominal rupture (prepubic tendon (3.71) or rectus abdominis muscle), hematoma, and severe udder edema (11.56).

Management: incurable condition. Moderate cases can often be kept for the remainder of the lactation, but are best housed in straw yards rather than cubicles (free stalls). Cluster attachment is often difficult due to teat displacement and the engorged udder. Breeding and prepartum overfeeding that leads to excessive udder engorgement are predisposing factors.

11

Infectious diseases

Introduction

Infectious diseases are a major limiting factor in cattle production in many parts of the world. In tropical Africa, with its 160 million cattle, the major diseases, i.e., rinderpest, foot-and-mouth disease (FMD), contagious bovine pleuropneumonia, theileriosis, and trypano-somiasis, are all infectious. Such limitations on livestock production lead to shortages of meat, milk, draught animals, and manure, and to the necessity to import from developed countries such as North America and Australia, and the European Union. These imports in turn discourage domestic livestock production, whilst the presence of infectious diseases bars the export of cattle and cattle products to developed countries.

Several infectious diseases have been covered and illustrated in earlier chapters.

Viral diseases

Several major bovine diseases, endemic in many parts of the world, have a viral etiology. They are characterized by their highly contagious nature and the variety of their cloven-footed hosts. Early recognition of suspicious signs and confirmation of the disease in the laboratory, together with prompt and effective control measures, are essential for their eradication.

Foot-and-mouth disease (FMD)

Definition: a highly infectious disease with a short incubation period caused by aphthovirus of the family *Picornaviridae* with seven serotypes. A transboundary disease of the OIE.

Clinical features: cattle infected with foot-and-mouth disease are dull, off feed, and drool saliva (12.1). Some are lame. On opening the mouth (12.2), large areas of epithelial loss, that are the result of recently ruptured FMD vesicles, are seen on the tongue and hard palate, as in this animal from Zimbabwe. 12.3 also shows recently ruptured tongue vesicles. An unruptured vesicle on the dorsum of the tongue is seen in 12.4.

In a steer infected experimentally, within 2 days initial vesicles have ruptured to reveal ulcers which are seen

12.1. FMD drooling

12.2. Foot-and-mouth disease (FMD): extensive loss of epithelium from tongue and gum (Zimbabwe)

12.4. FMD: unruptured tongue vesicle (approx. 24 hours)

12.5. FMD: ulcers on gums, inside lower lip and tongue (approx. 2 days)

along the lower gums and inside the lower lip, together with ruptured tongue vesicles (12.5). Two days later the lesions on the tongue, lower lip, and gums have become secondarily infected (12.6). Elsewhere a vesicle on the coronary band and dorsal part of the interdigital space has ruptured. On the seventh day (12.7) the interdigital space shows widespread ulceration along its entire length. A vesicle on the soft skin above the heel has ruptured in another cow (12.8). Lameness may be the first sign of

FMD. These interdigital lesions easily become secondarily infected. Multiple teat vesicles are shown in 11.28 (p. 211).

Differential diagnosis: includes vesicular stomatitis (4.11), BVD/MD (4.3), bovine papular stomatitis (4.13,

12.3. FMD: ruptured vesicles

12.6. FMD: secondary infection of oral ulcers (approx. 4 days)

12

12.7. FMD: interdigital space with widespread ulceration (approx. 7 days)

12.9. Rinderpest ("cattle plague"): appearance of epizootic (Nigeria)

4.14), rinderpest (12.13), digital dermatitis (7.57–7.60), interdigital dermatitis (7.65).

Management: slaughter policy in FMD-free countries, and elsewhere isolation, quarantine, and ring vaccination where disease is endemic.

Rinderpest ("cattle plague")

Definition: infectious disease caused by a *Morbillivirus* having variable virulence and a wide ungulate host range.

Clinical features: virgin-soil epizootics (12.9), here in Nigeria, fulminate rapidly and frequently escalate into panzootics, whereas enzootic rinderpest spreads slowly, even inapparently, for months in immature and young adult stock free of maternally-derived antibodies.

Clinical diagnosis in fresh epizootics is relatively easy: after a prodromal onset of fever, illness is evident in 48 hours. Affected animals are restless and have dry muzzles and staring coats. Milk yields fall, respirations are shallow and rapid, visible mucous membranes are congested, whilst tears (12.10) and nasal fluids (12.11) flow profusely. The appetite is impaired and constipation develops.

12.8. FMD: ruptured skin vesicle above heel

12.10. Rinderpest: affected eye in epizootic outbreak

12

12.11. Rinderpest: nose with foul discharge in epizootic outbreak

12.13. Rinderpest: abraded erosive lesions on dental pad, tongue, and gum

The emergence of mucosal erosions 2–5 days later is the first sign suggestive of rinderpest: raised pinheads of necrotic epithelium reminiscent of oatmeal coat all visible mucous membranes, for example tongue and lips (12.12). They are readily abraded to reveal shallow erosions with a hemorrhagic layer of intact basal cells (12.13). The erosions enlarge and coalesce throughout the alimentary tract from the mouth and esophagus (12.14) to the rectum. Salivation is profuse. The affected cattle are now obviously sick, drink excessively, and pass soft feces. In 2–3 days the fever regresses and diarrhea starts. The brown, fluid feces contain necrotic debris streaked with blood. Dehydration is rapid and the frequent straining reveals the capillary stasis in the rectum known as zebra stripes (12.15). Breathing is labored and painful. Most cattle die within 6–12 days of the onset of overt illness. Pregnant cows abort during convalescence that lasts for months. In contrast, enzootic rinderpest is difficult to diagnose clinically. Adult cows are immune and passively immunize their sucking progeny, protecting them for up to 9 months; thereafter they are at risk. The clinical signs are muted, and often one or more of

12.14. Rinderpest: extensive erosion in esophagus

the cardinal features of the classic epizootic syndrome such as fever, erosions, mucopurulent nasal and ocular discharges, and diarrhea are absent. Most affected animals survive and suspicions of rinderpest are not roused. The illustrations are from Saudi Arabia, Yemen, and Nigeria.

Differential diagnosis: lesions are indistinguishable from those in BVD (4.3). Other similar diseases are FMD

12.12. Rinderpest: raised pinheads of necrotic epithelium ("oatmeal") on tongue and lips

12.15. Rinderpest: capillary stasis in rectum ("zebra stripes")

(12.1–12.8), IBR (5.2), and malignant catarrhal fever (12.20–12.22).

Management: the incidence of rinderpest has declined spectacularly following massive international vaccination campaigns financed by Europe and the USA, and organized in Africa and Asia by the Food and Agricultural Organization of the United Nations (FAO) and the Office International des Épizooties (OIE). Today, rinderpest has been eradicated from the whole world, apart from a residual focus in southern Somalia, where serosurveillance and vaccination are difficult, due to the lawless state of the country. Previously infected countries are actively following OIE regulations (it is a transboundary disease), maintaining eradication of rinderpest. Early recognition and notification of new outbreaks are vital.

Bluetongue (BTV)

Definition: disease is caused by an orbivirus with many serotypes and is transmitted by windborne midges (*Culicoides*).

Clinical features: while endemic on the African continent, where it is characterized mainly by inapparent infections, bluetongue is sporadic in many other parts of the world, including Eastern Europe and the Mediterranean basin. Spread of BTV to Western European countries (including the UK, the Netherlands, and Germany) occurred in 2007. In North America it is a mild clinical condition and differential diagnosis is difficult. Infection is more common than disease, which presents as a hyperemic, inappetant animal. Bluetongue causes initial hyperemia of the muzzle and lips, followed by inflammatory and erosive lesions. This Dutch Holstein animal (12.16) shows a mucopurulent nasal discharge,

12.17. Bluetongue: sloughed oral mucosa (Netherlands)

hyperemia of the muzzle, and early gum erosions. Necrotic areas may be seen in the gums in a 2-year-old heifer (12.17) where the mucosa behind the incisor teeth has either sloughed or shows white diphtheritic plaques. Note the excessive salivation, a result of discomfort and a reluctance to close the jaws. Changes in the hard palate (12.18) include extensive areas of ulceration which extend onto the dental pad. Some clinical cases of BTV show irregular superficial teat erosions (12.19). Stiffness and laminitis, with distal edema of all limbs, may sometimes be seen. Clinical lesions in cattle are allegedly mediated by an IgE hypersensitivity reaction. Diagnosis is by PCR and AGID assay and by virus isolation.

12.16. Bluetongue: mucopurulent nasal discharge, gum erosions (Netherlands)

12.18. Bluetongue: necrosis of hard palate (USA)

12

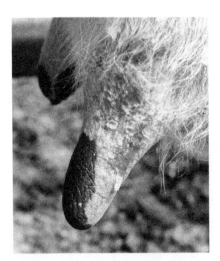

12.19. Bluetongue: superficial teat erosions

Differential diagnosis: photosensitization (3.4, 3.5), BVD (4.3), IBR (5.3), vesicular stomatitis (4.11), FMD (12.2).

Management: individual cases should receive supportive therapy. Vaccine is available for herds in epidemic areas. Attempt to reduce exposure to *Culicoides*.

Malignant catarrhal fever (MCF, bovine malignant catarrh, malignant head catarrh)

Definition: a worldwide sporadic, herpesvirus infection, almost invariably fatal. One (wildebeest-associated) form is caused by Alcephaline herpesvirus-1 (AHV-1), the other (sheep-associated) by ovine herpesvirus-2.

Clinical features: malignant catarrhal fever causes marked pyrexia, anorexia, and profound depression, with catarrhal and mucopurulent inflammation of the upper respiratory and alimentary epithelia, keratoconjunctivitis following a characteristic initial peripheral keratitis, and lymphadenopathy. Typically, a clinical case has a foul, pungent oral odor. MCF herd outbreaks are seasonal and occur predominantly in Africa. Elsewhere (North America and Europe), only sporadic cases are seen. The "head and eye" syndrome of the Devon cow in 12.20 includes a purulent oculonasal discharge, mild keratitis, and hyperemia of the nostrils. Note the almost pathognomonic hypopyon in the crossbred Charolais suckler cow in 12.21. There is a marked ocular discharge and pus is settling toward the base of the anterior chamber. Iridocyclitis may lead to photophobia. The nasal discharge is, unusually, not particularly severe. Areas of dry necrosis and ulceration are seen on the gums and dental pad of 12.22. Similar changes are commonly seen on the nostrils. Clinical cases in cattle are not infectious, but if they survive they are infected for life and may infect their calves *in utero*.

12.20. Malignant catarrhal fever (MCF): head and eye syndrome in cow (Devon)

Differential diagnosis: rinderpest (12.10, 12.11), bluetongue (12.16–12.19), East Coast fever (12.48), IBR (5.2), Schmallenberg virus (12.82), BVD/MD (4.1), Jembrana disease (Indonesia) (12.57–12.60), bovine iritis (8.36).

Diagnosis: by clinical picture, gross pathology, and confirmed in outbreaks by ELISA serology and PCR of viral DNA in host lymphocytes.

Management: despite occasional reports of success with cortisone and antibiotics, most cases are best culled as soon as the diagnosis is confirmed. Inactivated wildebeest-associated MCF vaccine is available in some countries. Some Western European countries have recently introduced voluntary vaccination programs. It is a transboundary disease of the OIE.

12.21. Malignant catarrhal fever: characteristic hypopyon in cow (Charolais cross)

12.22. Malignant catarrhal fever: dry necrosis and ulceration on gums and dental pad

Lumpy-skin disease (LSD)

Definition: a capripoxvirus disease of cattle first reported in Northern Rhodesia (Zambia) in 1929, now widespread in Africa, including Egypt, with recent spread into the Middle East. LSD affects European breeds of cattle most severely. Biting flies are the main vectors.

Clinical features: initially a fluctuating fever, lacrimation, and inappetance for 2 weeks, during which circumscribed nodules appear in the skin over the whole body (12.23) and mucous membranes of the mouth and respiratory tract, genitalia (orchitis), and conjunctiva. These nodules (12.24) are discrete, firm, raised, and painful, and contain hard gray-yellow material. Regional nodes

are enlarged (prescapular in 12.24). Edema of the lower limb is common in severely affected animals. Some nodules resolve rapidly, whilst others become firm necrotic sitfasts (12.23 body and 12.25 head and neck) that heal slowly and drop out, leaving a scar. Secondary infection can lead to suppurating ulcers and abscesses. A few nodules may persist for years. Subclinical cases develop isolated nodules which are often missed.

Mortality rates in endemic areas are 1–3%, but in virgin soil epizootics may approach 100%. In South Africa lumpy-skin disease is the most serious cause of economic loss in cattle, due to prolonged debility, milk loss, infertility in both cows and bulls, abortion, and hide damage.

Differential diagnosis: ulcerative lymphangitis (pseudotuberculosis) (3.48), pseudo-lumpy-skin disease (Allerton herpes virus infection) (12.26, 12.27), dermatophilosis (streptothricosis) (3.42).

Management: good nursing, sulfonamides or antibiotics for secondary infections, use of attenuated virus vaccine (Neethling strain). Slaughter policy of affected and contact cattle, coupled with vaccination of at-risk cattle before likely disease spread into a previously free area or country. It is a transboundary disease of the OIE.

Pseudo-lumpy-skin disease (LSD), (Allerton virus infection)

Definition: one of two bovine herpesvirus-2 syndromes (see also bovine herpes mammillitis, p. 208), pseudo (false)-lumpy-skin disease is characterized by transient moderate fever and exudative cutaneous plaques. Disease occurs primarily in southern Africa, and very occasionally in the USA, Australia, and the UK.

Clinical features: initial fever and mild lymphadenopathy are followed within a few days by emergence of numerous circular or oval superficial cutaneous plaques

12.23. Lumpy-skin disease (LSD): multiple skin nodules over trunk

12

12.24. Lumpy-skin disease: discrete nodules and enlarged prescapular nodules in cow (Jersey)

12.25. Lumpy-skin disease: resolution of some nodules with sitfast on face (Ethiopia)

about 1–2 cm diameter. These are hard, firm, have a red margin, and enlarge to 3–5 cm, becoming umbilicated. The centers are depressed and exude to form brown crusts (12.26). The skin beneath the crusts dies within 2 weeks to reveal smooth new skin, and fresh hair grows within 2 months. Lesions are frequently on the face, neck, back,

12.26. Pseudo-lumpy-skin disease: irregular cutaneous plaques over cheek and neck

12.27. Pseudo-lumpy-skin disease: multiple plagues, some brown and crusty in perineum and on udder skin (Charolais)

and perineum (12.27), as in this pedigree Charolais heifer in the UK. Clinical recovery is uncomplicated.

Diagnosis depends on clinical appearance and demonstration of herpesvirus-2 from peripheral lesions (skin scraping or punch biopsy). Biopsy will also reveal eosinophilic intranuclear inclusion bodies.

Differential diagnosis: lumpy-skin disease (12.24), urticaria (3.1, 3.2), dermatophilosis (3.37–3.43).

Management: nursing care.

Rift Valley fever (RVF)

Definition: acute febrile disease of cattle and sheep readily communicable to humans, and caused by a mosquito-borne phlebovirus (*Bunyaviridae*). Previously confined to Africa, including Egypt (1977–78), a major epidemic (2000) in Saudi Arabia and Yemen resulted in severe cattle losses and numerous human deaths.

Clinical features: calves usually die after a short peracute illness with high fever, severe dyspnea, and terminally lateral recumbency with extended legs and neck. Cows, following a transient fever, icterus, leucopenia, and incoordination, abort and may die. Nonpregnant adults experience a low-grade fever. Epidemics of RVF are linked to wet years in which hatching of larger numbers of infected mosquito eggs occurs (*Aedes linneatopennis*).

Autopsy changes in calves and fetuses include a spectacular bright orange-yellow and diffusely necrotic liver (12.28), whilst adult cattle show discrete focal necrotic hepatic lesions (12.29). Widespread hemorrhages are evident in the subcutaneous tissues, musculature, and serosa of the intestine (12.30). Diagnosis depends on viral isolation from aborted fetuses or blood. Veterinarians are at particular risk when handling infected tissues.

Differential diagnosis: ephemeral fever (12.31, 12.32), bluetongue (12.16–12.19), rinderpest (12.9), brucellosis ("storm").

12.28. Rift Valley fever (RVF): orange necrotic foci in liver of calf (Charolais)

12.29. RVF: diffuse focal hepatic lesions in adult cow

Management: control depends primarily on strict prohibition of the import of susceptible cattle and other species from endemic parts of the African continent and adjacent regions. Zoonotic spread from country to country by human carriers is possible. Attenuated killed virus and mutagen-attenuated vaccines are practical and economic control measures. It is a transboundary disease of the OIE.

12.30. RVF: subcutaneous and muscle hemorrhages

12.31. Ephemeral fever severe case in recumbent steer (South Africa)

Ephemeral fever ("three-day sickness")

Definition: an infectious, rarely fatal disease caused by a rhabdovirus transmitted by *Culicoides* (midges) and mosquitoes. Wind-borne dissemination occurs.

Clinical features: mild cases remain reasonably bright but are pyrexic, stiff, or slightly lame, and lactating cows have a pronounced drop in yield. Severe cases of ephemeral fever are initially seen in sternal recumbency and later in lateral recumbency (12.31) with signs of flaccid paralysis. Other features include rumen atony, loss of the swallow reflex and tongue tonus (12.32), and partial paralysis of the lower jaw (12.31), resembling botulism. Atypical interstitial pneumonia and lymphadenopathy may occur. Death is rare. The disease occurs in Africa, Asia, and Australia.

Differential diagnosis: botulism (2.69), pneumonia, severe toxemia, physical injury, Rift Valley fever (12.28), rabies (9.32–9.34).

Diagnosis: clinical signs and serology (CF, AGID, and ELISA).

12.32. Ephemeral fever: loss of tongue tonus and partial paralysis (South Africa)

12

Management: supportive care, e.g., NSAIDs and calcium solutions, may benefit recumbent cows. Prevention by annual vaccination and fly control.

Tick-borne diseases (protozoal and rickettsial infections)

In the tropics, ticks are very important owing to their impact on the cattle industry. Tick infestations depress productivity as a direct result of their feeding activity. This is primarily through reduced liveweight gain. Other consequences include anemia, skin wounds that are susceptible to secondary bacterial infection or screw-worm infestation (3.56), and toxic reactions to tick saliva (e.g., sweating sickness, 12.37). Indirectly, however, they have a far more significant role as vectors of diseases such as theilerioses that are widespread in subtropical Europe, Africa, and Asia.

Other tropical tick-borne diseases that limit cattle production include babesiosis, anaplasmosis, heartwater (cowdriosis), and dermatophilosis. Ticks parasitic on cattle can be divided into two families, the Ixodidae or "hard" ticks and the Argasidae or "soft" ticks, depending on the presence or absence of a hard, dorsal scutum. These families also have many other differences.

Tick infestations

Clinical features: taken in Antigua, West Indies, 12.33 shows *Amblyomma variegatum* (tropical African bont) ticks feeding on teats. These species are mainly found in the tropics and subtropics, causing disease both directly and by parasite transmission. Mixed tick infections do occur. Their large mouthparts can cause serious wounds that are liable to secondary infection. The scrotum is also a common region for tick feeding. In 12.34 *Amblyomma* species are seen in varying stages of engorgement, feeding around the perineum and anus of a 4-month-old Friesian heifer from Zimbabwe. White larvae along the edge of the tail indicate early myiasis lesions. These changes are more pronounced in 12.35, where tick damage has resulted in an enlarged vulva, with raw, bleeding areas. Early myiasis is again visible. Myiasis lesions are also shown in 3.56 and 3.57.

12.34. *A. variegatum* in various stages feeding around perineum and anus of heifer (Friesian, 4 months old) (Zimbabwe)

Cowdria ruminantium, the ehrlichial rickettsial agent of heartwater is carried by *A. variegatum*.

Diagnosis and management: see "Tick toxicosis," below.

Tick toxicosis

There are two distinct tick toxicoses: tick paralysis and sweating sickness.

Definition: tick paralysis is a widespread but sporadic affliction of calves induced by at least three tick species: *Ixodes* spp., *Dermacentor* spp., and *Haemaphysalis* spp. The toxin causes an ascending paralysis that spreads from the hind limbs to the fore limbs. Death follows respiratory failure.

12.33. Tick infestation involving teats: tropical African bont (*A. variegatum*)

12.35. Tick infestation: severe damage in enlarged bleeding vulva

12

12.36. Tick paralysis: recumbent heifers (France)

Sweating sickness is an acute noninfectious disease of calves caused by bites of female *Hyalomma* spp. ticks, whose saliva apparently contains an epitheliotropic toxin. The female *Hyalomma truncatum* appears to be infectious at a weight of 25–50 mg. The tick must feed for 5–7 days before sufficient toxin has entered the host calf.

Clinical features of tick paralysis: a flaccid paralysis is seen predominantly in calves and yearling cattle (12.36). These two crossbred heifers were unable to stand, dull, and anorexic. Ticks, primarily on the backs and flanks, were killed with insecticide spray, resulting in complete recovery in 4 days.

Clinical features of sweating sickness: it is seen in Central and Southern Africa and India. In the Friesian calf from Zimbabwe (12.37), the moist dermatitis (sweat) typically affects the inguinum, the perineum, and the axilla, producing a sour smell. Note the early myiasis ventral to the vulva. Young calves are usually affected and immunity lasts for 4–5 years. Hair loss, which may be total, occurs secondary to the initial moist dermatitis. Hair may be pulled off when the animal is handled, e.g., over the ears (12.38). Secondary skin infection often

12.38. Tick toxicosis: sweating sickness with secondary hair loss from ears (Zimbabwe)

develops. Lacrimation and salivation may occur because all mucous membranes are affected.

Diagnosis: demonstration of the vector tick. Differentials include cerebral babesiosis (12.39–12.41), cerebral theileriosis (12.48), meningitis (9.22, 9.23), encephalitis, rabies (9.33, 9.34).

Management: NSAIDs and broad-spectrum antibiotics to relieve dermatitis, and topical insecticides and acaricides to control secondary myiasis. Tick control to prevent further cases. In endemic areas cattle may have to be dipped weekly during the season of risk. No vaccine is available.

Babesiosis ("redwater fever", "Texas fever")

Definition: babesiosis covers a group of diseases carried by the protozoan *Babesia* spp., *B. bovis* and *B. divergens* being the most important, occurring singly or together and, combined with *Anaplasma*, can produce a fatal "tick fever". The major signs are fever and intravascular hemolysis, shown by anemia, hemoglobinuria and jaundice.

Clinical features: the South Devon cow in 12.39 has lost condition. She has a dejected appearance, with drooping ears, half-closed eyes, and the front legs abducted to maintain balance. Her flank is hollow, indicating lack of rumen fill. There is extreme pallor of the vulval mucosa as in 12.44, and the conjunctiva is both anemic and jaundiced (12.40). Dark, port-wine-colored urine, as seen in the South Devon steer in 12.41, often produces a characteristic golden-yellow froth as it hits the ground (12.42). Affected cattle are febrile and develop anal sphincter spasm, producing "coiling" of feces which are voided under pressure (12.43). Some animals may

12

12.37. Tick toxicosis: sweating sickness form with moist dermatitis ventrally in heifer (Friesian)

12.39. Babesiosis in dejected cow, poor condition, with half-closed eyes (South Devon)

12.42. Babesiosis: gold-colored, frothy urine

12.40. Babesiosis: anemic and jaundiced conjunctiva

die suddenly after 24 hours of acute illness, others may abort. *Ixodes ricinus* is the common vector for *Babesia bigemina*, the major form of babesiosis in the UK. Disease caused by babesiosis is distributed worldwide wherever there are ticks. In the tropics the most widespread and serious form of babesiosis is caused by *B. bovis*, transmitted by *Boophilus microplus*.

Differential diagnosis (of redwater): includes anaplasmosis (12.44), theileriosis (12.48), bracken poisoning (13.3), kale poisoning (13.10), leptospirosis in calves, bacillary hemoglobinuria, nitrate poisoning (13.27). Diagnosis is by examination of blood smear.

Management: individual treatment involves protozoal destruction by babesicides such as imidocarb

12

12.41. Babesiosis : dark, port-wine-colored urine in steer (South Devon)

12.43. Babesiosis: anal sphincter spasm and "coiled" feces

or amidocarb, and possibly blood transfusions in severe cases.

Prevention: eradication of ticks, (e.g., by pasture improvement), regular dipping, and possibly vaccination or chemoimmunization.

Tick-borne fever

Definition: a benign rickettsial disease caused by *Ehrlichia phagocytophila*, which parasitizes white blood cells. Tick-borne fever is limited to temperate regions of Europe, Africa and Asia. Natural tick vectors are *Ixodes ricinus* (Europe) and *Rhipicephalus haemophysaloides* (Asia), hence outbreaks are seasonal.

Clinical features: compared with babesiosis (p. 231) tick-borne fever is much less severe. Milking cows lose production and may abort, especially if recently introduced to the area. Cows are febrile, off feed, and appear stiff. Pregnant heifers in their second grazing season may experience a high fever ("pasture fever"), can cough, have drooping ears, and may abort. A depressed defense mechanism can result in secondary infection such as postparturient sepsis.

Differential diagnosis: babesiosis (12.39–12.42), brucellosis (10.89). Diagnosis is usually based on typical geographical location and tick activity. Giemsa-stained blood film 2–8 days after onset of fever can be diagnostic.

Management: avoid placing naïve heifers and cows in late pregnancy onto tick-infested pastures. Tetracyclines are effective in treatment and control.

Anaplasmosis ("gall sickness")

Definition: anaplasmosis is caused by a tick-borne ehrlichial parasite *Anaplasma marginale* which leads to disruption of host erythrocytes.

Clinical features: gall sickness is endemic in tropical and subtropical regions of Africa, Asia, Australia, and the Americas. Transmission is by ticks (*Boophilus* and *Dermacentor* spp.), biting flies, or iatrogenically, e.g., during mass vaccination. Calves infected remain infected throughout life. Most appear healthy, but if stressed will develop clinical signs. Adult cattle are more severely affected. After initial pyrexia and anorexia, anemia develops, as shown on the vaginal mucosa in 12.44, and later jaundice (12.45) of the vulvar mucosa. Hemoglobinuria is absent. In the occasional peracute case in a dairy cow severe pyrexia and dyspnea may be associated with hyperexcitability. Mortality may reach 50%.

On autopsy (12.46), the carcass is pale, anemic, and slightly jaundiced. Unclotted blood can be seen on the hide adjacent to the spine. The liver is enlarged and mottled (12.47), the distended gallbladder contains thick

12.44. Anaplasmosis: characteristic anemic vaginal mucosa

12.45. Anaplasmosis: jaundiced vulva

bile, and there is splenic enlargement. Recovered animals may remain carriers for life. (These illustrations are from Zimbabwe and from Queensland, Australia.)

Differential diagnosis: babesiosis (12.39–12.43), bacillary hemoglobinuria, theileriosis (12.48), trypanosomiasis (12.62). Diagnosis is on examination of a blood smear.

12.46. Anaplasmosis: carcass pale, anemic, slightly jaundiced (Zimbabwe)

12

12.47. Anaplasmosis: enlarged and mottled liver

Management: treatment is with tetracyclines or with imidocarb dipropionate, and possibly blood transfusion in very anemic cases. Prevention by insect control is not practical in many regions but an acaricide dip at weekly intervals in endemic areas controls ticks. Avoidance of iatrogenic transmission (syringes and needles). Vaccination regimes are currently controversial.

Theileriases

Definition: *Theileria* species are tick-borne protozoal parasites that multiply in lymphocytes and then enter erythrocytes.

Clinical features: theileriosis is common in tick-infested areas throughout the world. *T. parva* (East Coast fever, ECF), transmitted by *Rhipicephalus appendiculatus*, is a serious problem restricted to Central and East Africa. *T. annulata*, transmitted by *Hyalomma* species, occurs in North Africa, southern Europe, the Middle East, India, and Asia. Its pathogenicity varies but can result in mortality rates up to 90%. In 12.48, the Jersey heifer from Zimbabwe is in poor condition and shows gross enlargement of the parotid and prescapular lymph nodes, a rough coat (particularly dorsally), and matted hair over the face due to epiphora. Affected animals are pyrexic and anemic. On autopsy examination, splenic enlargement, severe pulmonary emphysema and edema, and generalized lymphoid hyperplasia are the most striking changes.

Differential diagnosis: trypanosomiasis (12.61, 12.62), cowdriosis (12.49–12.52), malignant catarrhal fever (12.20–12.22), contagious bovine pleuropneumonia (5.20–5.22).

Management: use of resistant cattle breeds, acaricides, vaccination (infection and treatment methods).

Cowdriosis ("heartwater")

Definition: caused by the ehrlichial rickettsia *Ehrlichia ruminantium* (formerly *Cowdria ruminantium*), heartwater is transmitted from reservoir wildlife hosts (e.g., wildebeest) to susceptible cattle by *Amblyomma* (bont) ticks, producing severe damage to the vascular endothelium, and results in pyrexia, hydropericardium, and nervous signs.

Clinical features: the disease is common in many parts of Africa and the Caribbean; the cattle illustrated are from Mali. Peracute disease produces rapid death. Acute cases are initially dull, pyrexic, anorexic, and diarrheic, with a "tucked-up" abdomen, as seen in the Zebu steer in 12.49. Nervous signs, convulsions, maniacal behavior, and death in extensor spasm may follow rapidly, with a frothy discharge from the nostrils (12.50). Increased vascular permeability produces a generalized circulatory failure, seen as lung congestion, hydrothorax, and hydropericardium (12.51, where the forceps raise the margin of the incised pericardium). In 12.52 the cut surface of an affected lung shows massive interlobular edema (A) and congestion (B). Disease is sometimes mild or inapparent.

Differential diagnosis: anthrax (12.63), rabies (9.33, 9.34), cerebral babesiosis (12.39), cerebral theileriosis

12.48. Theilerioses: poor condition and severe lymphadenopathy in heifer (Jersey) (Zimbabwe)

12.49. Cowdriosis ("heartwater"): dull, "tucked up" steer (Zebu) (Mali)

12.50. Cowdriosis: frothy nasal discharge in recumbent acute case

(12.48), meningitis (9.22, 9.23), enterotoxemia (*C. perfringens*, type D). Clinical signs in susceptible cattle (often imported) are usually diagnostic. Confirmation by demonstrating ehrlichial colonies in brain capillary endothelium.

Management: oxytetracyclines in clinical cases before the onset of clinical signs. Prevention by vaccination, tick control, and chemoprophylaxis.

Q fever

Definition: a worldwide zoonosis caused by *Coxiella burnetii*, a Gram-negative obligate intracellular parasite, which appears either as a small compact rod or large

12.52. Cowdriosis: massive pulmonary interlobular edema and congestion (South Africa)

pleomorphic organism inside vacuoles of the cytoplasm, causing abortion in cattle.

Clinical signs: infection is usually subclinical. Spread is by aerosol spray, direct contact, ingestion of infected placenta, or milk. Major risk is to pregnant women.

The uterus can develop a mild or severe placentitis. The organism can localize in the udder, drainage lymph nodes, placenta, and uterus, and can be shed at subsequent parturitions.

Differential diagnosis: other causes of abortion: diagnosis depends on demonstration of the organism (e.g., in placenta).

Management: need for treatment with tetracyclines rarely arises. Isolation of aborting cattle and destruction by burning of infected material (discharges, bedding) and aborted fetuses.

Sporadic bovine encephalomyelitis (SBE, "Buss disease", transmissible serositis)

Definition: SBE is caused by *Chlamydophila pecorum*. A recently described paramyxoviral SBE is a separate entity.

Clinical features: also known as transmissible serositis, it is an uncommon systemic infection with a

12.51. Cowdriosis: hydropericardium and lung congestion

12

12.53. Sporadic bovine encephalomyelitis: chronic fibrinous exudative peritonitis and pleurisy (South Africa)

worldwide sporadic distribution that causes a generalized inflammation of blood vessels, serous membranes, and synoviae. The calf in 12.53 shows a chronic fibrinous exudative peritonitis. Pleurisy and pericarditis were also present. The epidemiology and pathogenesis resemble MCF (12.20–12.22) but the mortality rate is low. Encephalitis develops secondarily to the mesenchymal damage.

Diagnosis: Giemsa-stained tissue impression smears, brain histopathology, or isolation of organism by tissue culture.

Differential diagnosis: bovine malignant catarrh, listeriosis (9.11, 9.12), rabies (9.32–9.34), lead poisoning (13.29), pneumonic pasteurellosis (5.8–5.11).

Management: possibly broad-spectrum antibiotics in early stages.

Bovine petechial fever (Ondiri disease)

Definition: the causal rickettsia is *Ehrlichia ondiri*. The natural mode of transmission is unknown but is likely to be a tick. The rickettsia is not contagious.

Clinical features: the organism is present in circulating granulocytes and monocytes during the clinical syndrome, and later localizes in the spleen and other organs. Disease is confined to altitudes above 1500 meters in Kenya and possibly neighboring Tanzania. Indigenous cattle do not develop clinical signs when infected. Newly arrived exotic cattle develop dramatic signs with sudden fever, which is often missed as cattle eat and behave normally. Dairy cows lose all milk production. Within 24 hours numerous petechiae develop in visible mucosae, e.g., beneath the tongue (12.54) as well as in internal organs such as epicardium (12.55) and the enlarged lymph nodes (12.56). Epistaxis, melena, and hyphema occur in severe cases. Hair follicles ooze blood and a straw-colored fluid which dries into a scurf. Scleral

12.54. Bovine petechial fever: petechiation below tongue (Zimbabwe)

and conjunctival hemorrhages may occur and occasionally free blood is present in the lower segment of the aqueous humor. The eyeball is tense, protruding through swollen, everted conjunctival sacs, as the so-called "poached egg eye." Snorting cattle trying to clear airways of blood and catarrhal exudate usually die, especially if pulmonary edema is present. The visible mucosae are white at death.

12.55. Bovine petechial fever: severe petechiation of epicardium (Zimbabwe)

12.56.   Bovine petechial fever: enlarged red lymph node contrasted with normal (Zimbabwe)

Diagnosis: demonstration of organisms in blood during febrile phase, typical history, and signs.

Management: systemic oxytetracycline in early stages of clinical disease. Recovered cases may remain latent carriers. Areas of previous outbreaks should ideally be avoided.

Jembrana disease

Definition: an immunosuppressive hemorrhagic diathesis of domesticated banteng (*Bos sondaicus* syn. *Bos javanicus*) in the Jembrana region on the island of Bali. Etiology is uncertain, possibly a *Boophilus* tick-borne ehrlichiosis, or a lentiviral infection (spread by close animal contact).

12.57.   Jembrana disease: Bali disease form with peripheral necrosis, e.g., ears (Indonesia)

Clinical features: first seen in 1964, when 61% of 31 000 banteng died, the disease has now spread to other Indonesian islands. Bali disease is another form, characterized by peripheral necrosis (e.g., ears 12.57) as a result of a generalized vasculitis. Early signs in virgin-soil epizootics include fever, anorexia, lethargy, and reluctance to move, as well as behavioral changes, severe generalized lymphadenopathy (12.58), and pallor. The cow shows enlarged parotid (A), retropharyngeal (B) and prescapular nodes (C). Feces may contain blood from intestinal hemorrhage (12.59). Pregnant animals may abort. Autopsy changes include severe hemorrhages in all organs including the hard and soft palate (12.60), and the serosal surface of the intestine. Proliferative changes are present in the lymphoreticular system, GI tract, liver, kidneys, and lungs. Endemic cases are milder and have about 20% mortality rate.

Differential diagnosis: rinderpest (12.10), hemorrhagic septicemia.

12.58.   Jembrana Bali disease showing severe lymphadenopathy (Indonesia)

12.59. Jembrana Bali disease: fecal blood following intestinal hemorrhage (Indonesia)

Management and control: recovered animals remain persistent carriers and are immune. There is considerable risk of disease transmission mechanically during mass vaccination against hemorrhagic septicemia. ELISA and AGID tests are available for survey work, but are not useful for diagnosis. Supportive treatment including tetracyclines may be helpful. No specific control is available.

Ehrlichiosis (Nofel syndrome)

Definition: *Ehrlichia bovis* is a persistent parasite of circulating monocytes of low pathogenicity in healthy cattle reared on tick-infested land where the parasite is endemic. Vectors are *Hyalomma aegypticus* (North Africa), *Amblyomma variegatum* (West Africa), *Rhipicephalus* (Southern Africa) and *A. cajennense* (Brazil).

Clinical features: naïve imports develop primary infection with fluctuating fever, anorexia, and diarrhea, lose condition, and may show nervous signs. Mortality is low. Another form (Nofel) is an exacerbated *E. bovis* infection in overstressed transhumant cattle which

develop marked lymphadenopathy, enormous edema in drooping ears, purulent oculonasal discharges, anorexia, and constipation. Most cattle die rapidly unless treated.

Differential diagnosis: cowdriosis (12.49–12.52).

Management: avoid introduction of susceptible naïve cattle, and practice regular dipping. Tetracyclines in severe cases.

Trypanosomiasis (African trypanosomiasis, Nagana)

Of all animal diseases, the most important constraint on animal production in the subhumid and humid tropics is trypanosomiasis, which in Africa alone affects animals in an area one-third larger than that of the USA. Annual losses may be as high as US$5 billion.

Definition: an acute, subacute, or chronic disease caused by blood parasites called trypanosomes. These are of various species: *Trypanosoma congolense* and *T. brucei* occur only in the areas of Africa where the vector, some 20 species of tsetse flies (*Glossina*), is found. *T. vivax* occurs not only in tsetse areas but also in the non-tsetse areas of Africa, Asia, and South and Central America. The parasites are cyclically transmitted biologically by tsetse but may be transferred mechanically during interrupted blood meals by other biting flies such as *Stomoxys*, *Tabanidae*, *Lyperosia*, and *Hippoboscidae*. The overwhelming majority of clinical infections of African trypanosomiasis are due to tsetse-transmitted *T. congolense* and *T. vivax*. *T. theileri*, a cosmopolitan species occurring in cattle, is nonpathogenic.

Clinical features: infection of cattle takes place through skin puncture and migration to the bloodstream via lymph nodes. The incubation period is 1–4 weeks. Clinical signs are nonspecific and include a staring coat, intermittent fever, dullness, anemia, lowered milk production, and loss of weight and condition (12.61, 12.62). Abortion and reproductive failure occur. There is a variable mortality rate although the chronic course may

12.60. Jembrana Bali disease: hemorrhages in hard and soft palates (Indonesia)

12.61. Trypanosomiasis: weight loss in group of grazing cattle

12.62. Trypanosomiasis: recumbent cow with severe weight loss

continue for months or years. There is also a peracute, hemorrhagic form associated particularly with strains of *T. vivax* in East Africa. Autopsy features are also nonspecific but include lymphadenopathy, depletion of fat, and anemia (pale and watery carcass). Hemorrhages may be seen in acute *T. vivax* cases as serosal lesions.

Diagnosis: livestock owners rely on clinical signs and response to treatment. Demonstration of parasites in stained blood and lymph gland smears or the centrifugation and examination of the buffy coat in fresh blood samples is definitive. The number of circulating parasites varies greatly so repeat sampling on an individual or herd basis may be necessary to demonstrate infection. Various serological tests involving immunological or molecular technology, which may indicate the degree of past exposure, are available.

Differential diagnosis: chronic wasting conditions such as fascioliasis, helminthiasis (e.g., schistosomiasis), babesiosis (12.39–12.43) anaplasmosis (12.44–12.47), East Coast fever (12.48), chronic CBPP, tuberculosis, malnutrition (energy, protein, or mineral deficiencies), and a combination of old age and repeated pregnancies. Acute hemorrhagic cases must be distinguished from hemorrhagic septicemia, bovine petechial fever, or Ondiri disease (12.54–12.56), and anthrax (12.63).

Management: treatment of clinical cases with diminazene aceturate (Berenil®), isometamidium (Samorin® or Trypamidium®), quinapyramine sulfate (Trypacide® and Triquin®), homidium bromide (Ethidium®), and homidium chloride (Novidium®). Drug resistance is an increasing problem.

Prevention: varying degrees of prophylaxis can be achieved by judicious use of isometamidium and homidium. Seasonal herding practices can reduce exposure to tsetse. Tsetse populations can be reduced by habitat modification and strategic application of insecticides to vegetation as pour-on formulations, or as dips and sprays to cattle, or on traps and insecticide-impregnated targets. Maintenance of trypanotolerant breeds, particularly the N'Dama and Muturu in West Africa is another strategy.

Bacterial diseases

Anthrax (splenic fever)

Definition: peracute disease caused by *Bacillus anthracis*.

Clinical features: most cases are seen as a sudden death in a previously healthy individual. A few cases in terminal septicemia are ataxic and have nasal, oral, or anal hemorrhage. Dark blood may be passed from anus and vulva terminally. The characteristic autopsy feature of anthrax is an enlarged, dark, soft-textured spleen, as seen in 12.63 in the specimen from a crossbred Hereford cow in Zimbabwe. Cattle may be infected through contaminated pastures (e.g., those flooded sporadically with river water carrying tannery effluent), or by eating contaminated artificial or natural feedstuffs. Cattle suspected as possible anthrax cases should not undergo autopsy examination, and diagnosis should be based initially on a blood smear. Anthrax is a notifiable disease in many countries. BSE regulations, which prohibit the feeding of meat and bone meal to cattle, have reduced the incidence of anthrax in the UK.

Differential diagnosis: other causes of sudden death, e.g., lightning strike (9.41), bloat (4.61, 4.62), clostridial diseases, (see below), anaplasmosis (12.44–12.47), bacillary hemoglobinuria.

Management: aggressive systemic penicillin or oxytetracycline therapy in early stages. Vaccination in endemic areas.

12.63. Anthrax: enlarged dark spleen in cow (Hereford cross Zimbabwe)

12

Clostridial diseases

Clostridia are natural inhabitants of the soil and of the gastrointestinal tract of humans and animals. Pathogenic effects in cattle arise either from ingestion or from wound contamination. One group of clostridia produces disease by active invasion and toxin production leading to death (tetanus, gas gangrene); the second produces toxins within the gut (enterotoxemia, caused by *C. sordellii*), or in food or carrion outside the body (botulism). One clostridial disease, malignant edema, caused by *C. septicum*, is illustrated in Chapter 4, "Alimentary disorders" (4.44, 4.45) to aid in differential diagnosis from other conditions leading to swelling of the head. A range of combined clostridial vaccines is widely available and very effective in preventing disease.

Blackleg (*Clostridium chauvoei*)

Definition: an acute febrile necrotizing myositis caused by *C. chauvoei*, characterized by emphysematous swelling.

Clinical features: blackleg develops spontaneously without a history of open wounds, although bruising may be a predisposing factor by producing anaerobic conditions in muscles that are harboring the organism. Occasionally fattening cattle are found dead without showing clinical signs. Most cases end fatally after signs of acute depression and lameness. The crossbred Charolais calf at pasture was severely lame with massive gluteal swelling of the right hind leg (12.64). Autopsy examination of the same animal (12.65) shows the blackened necrotic muscle compared with the normal left leg. The hindquarters usually have the most severe changes, seen as infiltration of the musculature with gas bubbles that have a characteristic rancid smell, although any part of the body, including heart muscle, may be affected. Often, severely affected muscle (dark) lies adjacent to normal tissue (12.65).

Differential diagnosis: malignant edema (4.45), anthrax (12.63), venomous snake bite, lightning strike

12.65. Blackleg: dark, necrotic, gluteal musculature (right), and normal (left)

(9.41–9.43). Gross pathological changes are usually characteristic, and laboratory confirmation is by fluorescent antibody staining.

Management: if not moribund, cattle may be treated with penicillin, NSAIDs, and possibly surgical debridement to expose surrounding tissues to atmospheric air. Vaccination on enzootic farms.

Tetanus (*Clostridium tetani*, "lockjaw")

Definition: tetanus toxemia is produced by a specific neurotoxin of *C. tetani*, usually as a disease passing up the nerve tracts to spinal cord and brain.

Clinical features: introduced into deep, anaerobic skin wounds (e.g., castration, 10.36), *C. tetani* causes progressive nervous signs as a result of neurotoxin production. Cattle show a generalized stiffness. The Hereford cross suckler cow (12.66) has an arched back and raised tail, extended head and neck, erect ears, "Chinese eyes," and flared nostrils. The third eyelid may be prolapsed. Ruminal bloat is common. This cow was hyperaggressive, then fell over and was unable to rise again. The disease progressed into severe extensor rigidity in a calf (12.67) with progressive respiratory failure. Rigidity is so severe that the upper feet remain off the ground. The tail is overextended. Note the severe opisthotonus. This calf had been castrated 2 weeks previously. A close-up view of a French cow (12.68) with tetanus demonstrates the muscular spasms in the stiff, extended neck, the caudally directed ears, and some feed, which cannot be masticated, between the paralyzed lips.

Differential diagnosis (in early cases): meningitis (9.24), cerebrocortical necrosis or polioencephalomalacia

12.64. Blackleg (*C. chauvoei*): massive swelling of the gluteal muscles in right hind leg (Charolais cross yearling)

12

12.66. Tetanus: arched back, extended head and neck, "Chinese eyes," and flared nostrils in cow (Hereford cross)

(9.1), hypomagnesemic tetany in calves (9.4), strychnine poisoning, acute muscle dystrophy (7.154).

Management: antisera, antibiotics, muscle relaxants, and supportive therapy in a quiet environment. Prevention by maintenance of proper skin and instrument disinfection at castration, and by vaccination.

Botulism (*Clostridium botulinum*, "Lamziekte")

Definition: a rapidly fatal motor paralysis, caused by a *C. botulinum* neurotoxin (usually type D).

Clinical features: the toxin is produced as a result of proliferation of the bacteria in decomposing animal matter, e.g., chicken manure spread onto pasture subsequently grazed by cattle or fed conserved forage from that pasture, or from carcasses of other birds and small mammals. The increase in cases in the UK may be due to withdrawal of in-feed antibiotic growth promoters. In the USA the majority of cases are associated with growth of *C. botulinum* in spoiled food, whereas in the UK poultry carcases, either from litter spread onto fields, ensiled or dragged onto grazing by foxes etc, is a common source. The toxemia results in initial posterior ataxia and progresses to paraparesis (12.69). The stance

may be straddled (base-wide) and the hind fetlocks may be knuckled. Motor paralysis of the tongue (12.70) causes difficulty in prehension, chewing, and swallowing. This cow could not hold its head up. Saliva may contain partially masticated feed material which cannot be swallowed. In the recumbent Angus cross cow the motor paralysis of the tongue is again evident

12.68. Tetanus: head and neck signs (France)

12.69. Botulism: posterior ataxia (USA)

12.67. Tetanus: marked extensor rigidity and opisthotonus

12

12.70. Botulism: motor paralysis of tongue in Friesian cow (USA)

12.71. Botulism in recumbent cow (Angus cross)

(12.71). In a large outbreak of botulism (fatalities 203/616 fattening stock) possibly due to consumption of vegetables in a mixed ration, a heifer collapsed onto slats in the cubicle house with severe respiratory distress (12.72). Note the extended head and neck, dilated nares, and open mouth. The tail is thrashing about. As in this

12.72. Botulism in collapsed beef heifer

outbreak, confirmation of *C. botulinum* is often impossible, either in sera, necropsy material, or suspect food. Death is from respiratory paralysis. In some countries the major cause of botulism is the ingestion of decomposed animal carcasses. This depraved appetite (pica) is stimulated by a phosphorus deficiency (7.164, 7.165). Up to 3% of cattle in endemic areas may die from botulism annually. Poultry manure (containing carcases) either spread onto pasture or used as cattle bedding, and in some countries ensiled poultry litter used as animal feed, have been implicated.

Differential diagnosis: organophosphorus toxicity (13.26), thromboembolic meningoencephalitis (9.27), BSE (9.36–9.38), SBE (12.53), paralytic rabies and trauma, listeriosis, postparturient paresis.

Management: correction of dietary deficiency, removal of source material, possibly immunization in problem areas with types D and/or C toxoid.

Mycoplasma wenyonii infection

Definition: *Mycoplasma* (formerly *Eperythrozoon*) *wenyonii* has recently been identified in Europe (UK) as a bovine pathogen affecting various body systems, but not involving the respiratory tract.

Clinical features: incidents, usually in late summer to autumn, have involved several dairy herds in which cows have suddenly developed a bilateral hindlimb edematous swelling (12.73) as well as teat and udder edema. Cows experience a sudden drop in yield, are anorexic, pyrexic, and have enlarged lymph nodes. Mycoplasma haemobos may be the cause of the sudden onset single quarter oedema syndrome in mid lactation cows.

Differential diagnosis: traumatic damage to hindquarters, circulatory failure (right heart), salt imbalance, or toxicity.

Management: general fly control measures. Avoidance of use of a single needle for multiple injections into several animals. Treatment with tylosin has been encouraging.

Miscellaneous

Bovine leukosis (bovine viral leukosis, bovine lymphosarcoma)

Leukosis occurs in four forms. The calfhood, thymic, and skin types are all termed sporadic leukosis. Bovine leukosis virus cannot be cultured from, nor antibodies be detected in, these three forms. The fourth type, the adult form, is known as enzootic bovine leukosis (EBL) and is caused by the bovine leukosis virus (BLV).

Calfhood multicentric lymphosarcoma

The Guernsey calf in 12.74 showed generalized lymphadenopathy with gross symmetrical enlargement of the

12.75. Thymic lymphosarcoma: presternal mass in heifer (Guernsey)

prescapular, submandibular, parotid, and retropharyngeal nodes. Palpation revealed that the lymph nodes were smooth, painless, and freely moveable, not involving the skin. Widespread tumor metastases are present in such cases, usually <6 months old. Like other forms of bovine leukosis, calfhood leukosis has a low and sporadic incidence.

Thymic lymphosarcoma

A large, firm, smooth mass is present in the presternal region of the yearling Guernsey heifer in 12.75. Edema is also present. Most cases are seen in the 6–24 months age group. Generalized lymphadenopathy was absent. Some cases have bloat as a result of esophageal obstruction. As in the multicentric form, a cross-section (12.76) of the discrete tumor from a 15-month-old crossbred Angus reveals pale yellow material without granulomatous contents.

Skin lymphosarcoma

Skin leukosis is rare and is seen in immature animals aged 6–24 months. The yearling steer in 12.77 has

12.73 Mycoplasma wenyonii: note edematous swelling of right hock compared to normal leg on left

12.74. Calfhood multicentric lymphosarcoma: gross symmetrical lymphadenopathy in calf (Guernsey)

12.76. Thymic lymphosarcoma: cross-section of mass (Angus crossbred, 15 months old)

12

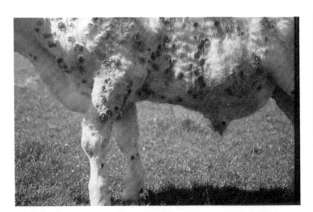

12.77. Skin lymphosarcoma with gray-white nodules

12.79. EBL: generalized lymphadenopathy in lymphosarcoma

gray-white nodules over the neck, back, flanks, and fore-limbs, which extend deep into the subcutis. There is also a generalized lymphadenopathy with prominent precrural nodes. In 12.78 another animal has skin leukosis limited to large, ulcerated lesions around the head. This is the only nonfatal lymphoid tumor in cattle, and these cutaneous masses regress after some months.

Differential diagnosis: actinobacillosis (4.37), actinomycosis (4.40), fibropapillomata (warts) (3.44).

Enzootic (adult) bovine leukosis (EBL), bovine lymphosarcoma

Definition: fatal systemic malignant neoplasia of reticuloendothelial system caused by an exogenous C-type oncovirus (BLV).

Clinical features: enzootic bovine leukosis produces a generalized lymphadenopathy with symmetrical enlargement of most peripheral nodes, often with other signs (12.79). The Angus cow in 12.80 had enlarged submandibular, parotid (shaved for needle biopsy before photography), and prescapular nodes. Lymphosarcoma was also found in the heart and uterus. Some cases (20%) have a predilection, usually unilateral, for the orbit. The

12.80. Enzootic bovine leukosis (EBL): generalized lymphadenopathy in cow (Angus)

12.78. Skin lymphosarcoma: large ulcerated masses around head

12.81. Bovine lymphosarcoma: bilateral retrobulbar masses causing exophthalmos in cow (Friesian) (USA)

neoplasia is generally retrobulbar. Exceptionally, the adult cow in 12.81 has massive bilateral exophthalmos and protrusion of granulation tissue as a result of lymphomatous infiltration into the orbit. Other sites of lymphosarcoma include the globe itself (8.42), the spinal canal and cord, causing progressive posterior paresis as a result of spinal cord compression (7.81), and the abomasum (4.75).

Differential diagnosis of EBL: sporadic bovine leukosis, traumatic pericarditis and congestive heart failure, lymphadenitis due to TB or actinobacillosis.

Diagnosis: histological examination of enlarged node.

Management: serological testing of herd at 3-month intervals and culling of positive cases.

Schmallenberg virus (SBV)

Definition: emerging disease identified in Germany in 2011 and now spread widely in Europe, including the UK and Ireland. Caused by an Orthobunyavirus in cattle, sheep and goats, SBV is not considered to be of major significance.

Clinical features: several cattle in a herd show fever, reduced milk yield, inappetance and perhaps diarrhea, recovering after a few days, although many herds become strongly seropositive without any apparent clinical signs. Pregnant cattle may abort or produce calves with arthrogryposis (12.82), jaw deformities, paralysis, hydrancephaly or torticollis (1.15). SBV appears to be transmitted by midges, although the rate of spread is so rapid that it suggests other routes may be involved.

12.82. Fetus affected with Schmallenberg virus (GD Deventer, Netherlands)

Differential diagnosis: Akabane virus (1.12), complex vertebral malformation (CVM) gene (p. 5), dwarfism (p. 2), or other causes of abortion (p. 199), winter dysentery (p. 58), bluetongue (p. 225) as midge-transmitted disease.

Diagnosis: serological screening by bulk milk antibody or individual animal bloods; confirmed by PCR for viral DNA from fetal material.

Management: a vaccine is currently (January 2013) in production, but until factors such as persistence of immunity following natural infection and the rate of exposure of heifers within an endemically infected herd are known, it is difficult to advise on its use. Careful foetal palpation in dystocia cases in known infected herds. No trade restrictions are currently in place.

12

Toxicological disorders

Introduction

Illustrations of toxicological disorders in cattle present problems. The clinical signs may be transient, with death occurring within a few minutes, such as in yew (*Taxus baccata*) poisoning (p. 249). In many cases the signs may be nonspecific. Where the effects are confined largely to one system, the description has been given in the appropriate section, e.g., ergot and fescue foot are considered under locomotor disorders (7.158–7.160). In this chapter, toxicoses have been broadly grouped into plant, organic, and inorganic chemical sections, and a few examples are given of each group. They are taken from Brazil, China, Germany, New Zealand, South Africa, the UK, the USA, and Zimbabwe.

Food safety issues arising from residues of chemicals in meat, offal, and milk are extremely important. Farmers are obliged, under food safety regulations, to avoid contaminating the food chain and must withdraw produce contaminated with chemical residues from the food chain. Food businesses such as dairies and supermarkets will reject produce from farms with unresolved poisoning incidents.

Plant toxicoses

Bracken (bracken fern)

Definition: acute or chronic worldwide toxicity following ingestion of large quantities of bracken (bracken fern), which contains several bone marrow toxins (aplastic anemia factor) which kill precursor cells in the bone marrow.

Clinical features: bracken toxicosis is widespread in several continents. Bracken (*Pteridium aquilinum*) contains ptaquilosides and other compounds which act as a cumulative poison in two syndromes. Firstly, after ingesting large quantities for a few weeks, cattle may show an acute syndrome resulting from aplastic anemia and thrombocytopenia. Sudden death is occasionally seen. In 13.1 the vulva of the crossbred Angus cow is pale from severe anemia. The pinpoint hemorrhages result from thrombocytopenia. Hemorrhages elsewhere can cause epistaxis, hyphema (13.2) (bleeding into the anterior chamber), or hematuria from bladder mucosal hemorrhage (13.3).

Secondly, long-term ingestion of considerable quantities of bracken for several months can lead to a chronic syndrome of enzootic hematuria. The ptaquilosides are carcinogens and cause bladder neoplasia, resulting in enzootic hematuria and malignancies such as hemangiosarcoma (13.4). Numerous discrete masses, seen protruding from the mucosal surface, bleed readily as the bladder distends and contracts. Some mucosal areas (top right, lower left) appear normal. The hemangiomata can develop into ulcerating tumors of various types. Alimentary tract neoplasms include squamous cell carcinomas and papillomas affecting the pharynx and esophagus, respectively. 13.5 shows pharyngeal squamous cell carcinomas (A) and esophageal papillomas (B) identified in Brazil. Bovine papillomavirus (types 2 and 4) may also be involved in upper alimentary neoplasms.

13.1. Bracken poisoning: pale vulvar mucosa in cow (Angus cross)

13.2. Bracken poisoning: hemorrhages causing hyphema

Differential diagnosis: acute syndrome: anthrax (12.63), septicemic pasteurellosis (5.10), PPH syndrome (9.39), mycotoxicosis (p. 253); chronic cases: pyelonephritis (10.1, 10.2), cystitis, babesiosis (12.41).

Diagnosis: a history of exposure to bracken, clinical signs of severe anemia and pancytopenia, and low platelet counts. Most outbreaks in grazing cattle have many

13.4. Bracken poisoning: several hemangiosarcomata protruding from bladder mucosa

subclinically affected animals with markedly abnormal blood parameters.

Management: treatment of individual cases is usually hopeless, possibly blood transfusion (5–10 liters); pasture and grazing management (bracken eradication). Food safety implications, resulting from the excretion of bone marrow toxins into milk, have led to the recommendation of a 4-day withdrawal period (UK) before milk can be consumed directly from bracken-grazed dairy cows.

Oak (acorn)

Definition: oak (*Quercus* species) containing a gallotannin, may cause toxic signs following several days' subacute ingestion of acorns (autumn) or young leaves (spring).

Clinical features: the toxic principle causes renal and gastrointestinal changes. The signs include abdominal pain, often with a hemorrhagic diarrhea, thirst, polyuria, and ventral edema as a result of subacute and chronic toxicity. The esophageal mucosa can be hemorrhagic (13.6). The enlarged, swollen kidneys (13.7) show scattered hemorrhages and a nephrosis, which accounts for the ventral edema, ascites, and hydrothorax seen in cases with renal failure.

13

13.3. Bracken poisoning: bladder mucosal hemorrhage

13.5. Bracken poisoning: alimentary tract neoplasis: (A) pharyngeal squamous cell carcinomas, (B) esophageal papillomas (Brazil)

13.6. Oak (acorn) poisoning: hemorrhagic esophageal mucosa

13.8. Yew poisoning: opened rumen with yew leaves

Diagnosis: history of known access to young oak leaves or acorns; autopsy features.

Management: symptomatic treatment (NSAIDs and fluid therapy). Prevent sudden access to acorns, e.g., following violent storms.

Yew

Definition: yew (e.g., *Taxus baccata*—English yew, *T. cuspidata*—Japanese yew) contains a cardiotoxic alkaloid, taxine, as well as cyanide.

Clinical features: signs usually follow acute exposure and include nervousness, ataxia, dyspnea, and collapse. The opened rumen in 13.8 shows normal ingesta mixed with needle-like yew leaves. Cattle usually die minutes after ingesting a few mouthfuls of yew twigs or berries, typically encountered as fresh or dried clippings thrown over a graveyard hedge into a bare winter pasture. The lethal dose in adult cattle may be as little as 1 kg of leaves. Some cattle may survive up to 3 days before they die.

Management: oral B$_{12}$, sucrose and also atropine have been suggested for treatment. Emergency rumenotomy may be considered for valuable animals.

Ragwort (seneciosis)

Definition: *Senecio jacobea* is one of many species of ragwort worldwide which contain the pyrrolizidine alkaloid jacobine, that causes acute and more often chronic liver disease. Several other plants e.g. *Crotalaria*, contain similar pyrrolizidine alkaloids which also can result in chronic hepatotoxicity.

Clinical features: early signs include dark-colored diarrhea, photosensitization, jaundice, abdominal pain, and central nervous system abnormalities. Prolonged ingestion (chronic exposure) results in progressive weakness, weight loss, and liver failure due to cirrhosis, and severe lung disease. In the mature Hereford cow in 13.9, the resulting right heart failure led to the edema affecting the ventral body wall, brisket, and head. Clinical signs may not be seen until several months after digestion, by which time the animal is no longer

13.7. Oak poisoning: enlarged swollen kidneys with multiple hemorrhages

13.9. Ragwort poisoning (seneciosis): ventral edema of abdomen, brisket, and head

13

consuming the toxin, and diagnosis can be difficult. Liver biopsy may be useful for diagnosis. The fresh plant is bitter and usually avoided. Intoxication frequently occurs following its incorporation into conserved forage as this renders the plant more palatable. See also photosensitization (p. 30).

Differential diagnosis: mycotoxicosis (p. 253), lead poisoning (13.29), and other causes of hepatic disease and encephalopathy.

Management: no useful treatment for pyrrolizidine alkaloid toxicity. Remove clinically normal cattle to uncontaminated food supply. Avoid making hay or silage from ragwort-infested pastures, especially in late summer and autumn.

Rape and kale

Definition: some forms of forage of the *Brassica* family, such as kale and rape, contain glucosinolates which with plant myrosinase can be hydrolyzed to S-methylcysteine sulfoxide (SMCO) which can cause a hemolytic (Heinz-Ehrlich body) anemia following production of dimethyl disulfide by ruminal bacteria. The flowers and seeds of mature plants are particularly poisonous, whether ingested by grazing cattle or in cake or meal. Glucosinolates cause goiter, encephalomalacia ("rape blindness"), pulmonary edema, and interstitial pneumonia.

Clinical features: cattle develop hemoglobinuria, voiding dark-red urine (13.10), and are anemic and weak. Autopsy of fatal cases reveals pallor and jaundice of the liver (13.11) and heart (13.12).

13.11. Rape and kale poisoning: pale jaundiced liver (USA)

Differential diagnosis: postparturient hemoglobinuria (possibly related to SMCO via a cumulative effect in red cells), bacillary hemoglobinuria, nitrate/nitrite poisoning (13.27, 13.28), hypomagnesemia (9.5), babesiosis (12.39–12.43), anaplasmosis (12.44–12.47), acute bracken poisoning (13.1–13.3), chronic copper poisoning (13.33).

Management: clinical signs are seen only following prolonged high intakes, e.g., 40–50 kg per day. Provide ample hay. Treat symptomatically for anemia. Switch to double zero rape strains to avoid toxicity.

Lantana

Definition: *Lantana camara* is a shrub containing toxic triterpenes which cause hepatic degeneration in cattle, producing signs of photosensitization, jaundice, rumen stasis, and depression.

13.10. Rape and kale poisoning: passage of dark red urine (hemoglobinuria) (USA)

13.12. Rape and kale poisoning: pale jaundiced heart (USA)

13

13.13. *Lantana* poisoning: severe photosensitization, depression, and tenesmus in steer (Holstein) (Zimbabwe)

13.14. *Solanum malacoxylon* toxicity: emaciation and stiffness in cow (crossbred) (Brazil)

Clinical features: in 13.13 the Holstein steer from Zimbabwe shows severe skin lesions (typical of photosensitization in that only the white areas are affected), depression, and tenesmus resulting from constipation. See also Chapter 3, photosensitization (p. 30), and facial eczema (p. 253).

Differential diagnosis: photosensitization (3.3–3.9), facial eczema (13.22–13.24).

Management: avoid access. Unless seen in the early stages of skin edema, treatment (e.g., with NSAIDs) is of limited value and the skin slough will run its course.

Solanum malacoxylon and *Trisetum flavescens* (enzootic calcinosis, enteque seco, Naalehu, espichamento)

Definition: *Solanum malacoxylon* (syn. *Solanum glaucophyllum*) (South America) or *Trisetum flavescens* (yellow oat grass) (Bavaria) acts by increasing calcium absorption from the gut through a glycoside of 1,25-dihydroxycholecalciferol (or a very similar compound). The glycoside is hydrolyzed by digestion, releasing the active vitamin D, and leading to a chronic syndrome of excessive deposition of periosteal new bone and calcification of blood vessels with progressive stiffness, lameness, and resulting weight loss.

Clinical features: this periosteal new bone and vascular calcification may be appreciated on rectal palpation (aorta) and on the lower limb (distal arteries). In 13.14 the crossbred cow from Mato Grosso, Brazil, is typically emaciated, stiff, and stands on the toes of the forefeet. Walking was typically slow and awkward. The endocardium and lungs of another cow (13.15) have areas of calcification (A), and the lungs have patches of ossified tissue (B). Calcification of the deep flexor tendons and

13.15. *Solanum malacoxylon* toxicity: (A) endocardial calcification, (B) pulmonary calcification (Brazil)

blood vessels is present in this German cow (13.16) with *T. flavescens* toxicity.

Other *Solanum* species can cause cerebellar degeneration or "crazy cow syndrome" in the USA. The nightshade group (e.g., *Solanum nigrum*, black nightshade) can produce gastrointestinal irritation and nervous signs.

13.16. *Trisetum flavescens* toxicity: calcification of deep flexor tendon and vessels (Germany)

13

13.17. *Tetrapteris* toxicity: ventral edema and depression in cow (Zebu cross, 5 years old) (Brazil)

Diagnosis: may be difficult in the early stages. Later signs and autopsy evidence of calcification of soft tissues (heart, major vessels, pleura, lungs) is diagnostic.

Management: removal from affected pasture, if feasible.

Tetrapteris species (peito inchado)

Definition: *Tetrapteris* species (*T. multiglandulosa* and *T. acutifolia*) cause a widespread cardiomyopathy in south-eastern Brazil.

Clinical features: cattle develop ventral, especially brisket, edema (hence peito inchado or swollen breast), jugular venous distension, and cardiac arrhythmia, as seen in a 5-year-old crossbred Zebu cow (13.17). The disease, usually subacute, is sometimes chronic, but rarely peracute. Autopsy lesions include myocardial pallor with some whitish streaking, and increased firmness suggestive of fibrosis, as seen in another mature Zebu cow in 13.18. *Tetrapteris* poisoning has been reproduced by feeding fresh or dry plant material for 9–50 days. The same plant may be responsible for stillbirths.

Selenium toxicity (locoweed, selenosis)

Definition: enzootic disease resulting from toxic amounts of selenium incorporated in specific ("converter") plants.

Clinical features: occasionally, as a result of careless selenium supplementation, acute selenium poisoning occurs and causes diarrhea, dyspnea, and death. Such supplementation may be as medication or a feed additive, e.g., together with an anthelmintic or currently with monensin. The problem is the narrow safety margin (1:10) between minimal requirement and toxic dose.

Enzootic selenosis occurs in specific areas of North America, Ireland, Canada, Israel, Australia, and South Africa where the soils contain a high level of selenium. Clinical signs, which are similar to swainsonine toxicity (13.19), include emaciation, hair loss, and claw deformities, resulting from prolonged ingestion of excessive selenium (exceeding 5 ppm in diet) incorporated in *Astragalus* species, which are selenium accumulator plants. A horizontal band starts below the coronary band and moves slowly distally. Pain, producing severe lameness, results from the movement of wall horn over the exposed sensitive laminae (13.20). Affected cattle may be forced to graze in a kneeling position. Another toxic syndrome is "blind staggers." Other toxins can also contribute to the clinical picture.

Differential diagnosis: diagnosis is based on clinical signs, autopsy, and laboratory evidence of high selenium levels in diet. "Blind staggers," previously considered etiologically a form of selenium toxicity, is now attributed to a excessive sulfate rather than selenium.

Management: elimination of source, symptomatic support. Follow manufacturer's advice on dose rates!

13.18. *Tetrapteris* toxicity: cardiomyopathy with myocardial pallor and fibrosis in cow (Zebu) (Brazil)

13.19. Selenium toxicity ("locoweed"): emaciation, hair loss, and claw deformities (USA)

13.20. Selenium toxicity: severe claw deformation (USA)

Lupine toxicity (crooked calf disease)

Definition: crooked calf disease is a generalized congenital defect caused by the neurogenic quinolizidine alkaloid anagyrine in *Lupinus caudatus* and *L. sericeus*, in some cases the alkaloid being in an *Aphis* on a lupine plant. Reduction of fetal movement is the cause of the teratogenic effects (e.g., joint contracture, torticollis, scoliosis).

Clinical signs: deformed calves, with variable degrees of malalignment of the long bones, are born to cows that have ingested large quantities of these lupine plants and *L. sericeus* during pregnancy. The calves in 13.21 were born to cows fed lupines from the 40th to the 70th day of gestation. Lupine species can also cause liver toxicity. See Chapter 1 (1.15) for other forms of arthrogryposis (e.g., BVD/MD virus infection).

Management: cows should not be grazed on lupine pastures during the period when they are liable to be 40–120 days pregnant.

Mycotoxicoses

Definition and clinical signs: mycotoxicosis is poisoning due to the ingestion of a fungal secondary metabolite. Seen chiefly in New Zealand, e.g., ryegrass staggers presents as an ataxia, initially in the hind legs, later progressing to the forelimbs and recumbency. The cause is the toxin lolitrem B, produced by the fungus *Acremonium lolii*, which is found in dry conditions in perennial ryegrass swards. Aflotoxicosis is another example where one or more systems may be affected to cause insidious effects such as reduced production and immunosuppression, or severe clinical disease with hepatic degeneration and tumors. Possible presentations include weight loss, depressed milk production, lower growth rates, abortion, lower limb swelling, skin changes, and nervous and other signs. Several other mycotoxins are immunosuppressants and could contribute to infectious disease. Zearalenone is an estrogenic compound, which affects fertility and induces premature mammary development.

Differential diagnosis: due to the wide range of clinical signs, no differentials have been listed. For example, lower limb swelling could be due to a wide range of physical, traumatic, metabolic, and/or infectious conditions.

The photomycotic dermatitis associated with the fungus *Pithomyces chartarum* is the selected illustrated example for description. Other examples of mycotoxicoses are illustrated in Chapter 7 (fescue foot, 7.158; ergot, 7.159, 7.160). Photosensitization is covered in Chapter 3 (3.3–3.9).

Facial eczema (pithomycotoxicosis)

Definition: photomycotic disease of grazing cattle caused by sporidesmins, which are secondary metabolites of a saprophytic fungus, *Pithomyces chartarum*.

Clinical signs: facial eczema is an economically important disease in New Zealand, and also occurs in Australia, France, South Africa, and South America. The fungus produces a hepatotoxic agent, which is commonly associated with ryegrass pastures. The clinical signs include lethargy, anorexia, conjunctivitis, jaundice, and a photosensitive dermatitis. At an early stage, the thin skin of the udder of

13.21. Lupine toxicity: two calves with severe long bone deformities (Hereford) (USA)

13

13.22. Facial eczema: hair loss and moist dermatitis of udder in (Jersey) cow (New Zealand)

13.24. Facial eczema: extensive photodermatitis in calf (Zebu, 1 month old) (Brazil)

the Jersey cow in 13.22 had lost its hair, and a moist dermatitis and hyperemia were evident. The skin in the upper left denuded area was starting to slough and the teats were also involved. Affected cows may lick this area of mild chronic irritation.

A late stage of facial eczema (13.23) shows a Friesian heifer with an extensive skin slough, typically confined to the white area. Note the involvement of the forelimbs (A), where carpal flexion has caused sloughing, and the thickened, wrinkled appearance of the skin extending down the hind legs (B). In a Brazilian Zebu herd, a 1-month-old male calf (13.24) had an extensive photo-dermatitis involving the ventral neck fold and chest wall and flank. The same fungus, *Pithomyces chartarum*, was consumed by the dam from a pasture of *Brachiaria decubens*, sporidesmin being ingested through the milk. The dam is normal.

Differential diagnosis: other forms of photodermatitis. Exposure to ryegrass, sunshine, typical signs, and characteristic appearance of the liver are pathognomonic.

Management: avoidance of exposure at critical times, pasture control such as sowing clover, alternating grazing, and use of fungicidal sprays to reduce the build-up of *P. chartarum* spores. NSAIDs may be helpful in early stages. Prevention by zinc supplementation (beware toxicity) via drench of zinc oxide, pasture application, or in drinking water.

Organic toxicoses
Chlorinated naphthalenes

Definition: naphthalenes, formerly extensively used as lubricants and wood-preserving compounds, are agents that cause hypovitaminosis A by interfering with the conversion of carotene to vitamin A.

Clinical features: hyperkeratosis of skin, emaciation, and possibly death result when naphthalenes are ingested over a long period. In 13.25 the head of the South African Friesian cow shows thickening, scaliness, and wrinkling of the skin. The hindquarters also had severe changes over the gaskin, hock, and metatarsus.

13.23. Facial eczema: extensive skin loss in trunk and forelimbs in heifer (Friesian) (New Zealand)

13.25. Chlorinated naphthalene toxicosis: hyperkeratosis of skin of head in cow (Friesian) (South Africa)

13

13.26. Carbonate toxicity: semicomatose hypersalivating cow (Angus cross) (USA)

Carbamate and organophosphorus compounds

Definition: these organophosphates inactivate cholinesterase, causing a rise in tissue acetylcholine and increased parasympathetic activity.

Clinical features: since the toxic signs of carbamate and organophosphorus tend to be similar, both organic groups can be discussed together. Poisoning is relatively common. The source of the toxin may be recently-sprayed orchards, cereal crops or hay, or excessively high concentrations in topical spray ("pour-on") preparations, although in most countries the use of the latter is no longer permitted. Major signs are salivation, lacrimation, urination, diarrhea, muscle tremors, and pupillary constriction in acute cases.

The crossbred Angus cow in 13.26 had ingested a carbamate insecticide powder (carbofuran or Furadan) from a half-empty bag about 6–16 hours previously. Initial generalized muscle twitching, depression, and locomotor incoordination were accompanied by hypersalivation. The cow then became semicomatose. Still salivating profusely, she showed miosis, severe dyspnea and pronounced bradycardia, and died 2 hours later. Her calf (13.26) was healthy throughout.

Differential diagnosis: nitrate and gyanide poisoning (13.27), acute grain overload (4.56), acute interstitial pneumonia or "fog fever" (5.28), acute anaphylaxis, urea toxicity.

Diagnosis: exposure to agent in feed or environment.

Management: in early acute disease massive doses of atropine (0.25 mg/kg) and possibly also oximes. Avoid use in stressed and sick stock.

Inorganic chemical toxicoses

Nitrate/nitrite

Definition: nitrates form nitrites before or after ingestion, and cause respiratory distress because methemoglobin formation leads to an anoxic anemia.

13.27. Nitrate/nitrite toxicity: congested red-brown vaginal mucosa (Netherlands)

Clinical signs: nitrites are about ten times as toxic as nitrates. The sources of nitrate/nitrite are numerous and variable in type, and include cereals, certain weeds (e.g., thistles, docks, Johnson grass), specific plants, and both organic and inorganic fertilizers. Apart from the predominant sign of dyspnea, muscle tremors and weakness with stumbling may be seen. In some outbreaks abortion may occur a few days later. A characteristic feature of this type of poisoning (nitrate/nitrite, also chlorate and metal ions (copper)) is the brown color of the vaginal and other mucosa and blood. Levels of 22% (13.27) and 60% (13.28) methemoglobinemia are illustrated. Clinical signs include tachypnea, muscle tremors, and ataxia. They appear at a level of about 20% conversion of hemoglobin to methemoglobin, while death follows at 60–80%.

Differential diagnosis: silo gas (nitrogen dioxide), hydrogen sulfide poisoning from underfloor slurry systems, sodium chlorate poisoning, acute rape or kale toxicity (13.10–13.12), and cyanide (bright-red oxygenated blood at autopsy), carbon dioxide (cyanosis), cobalt, or chronic copper poisoning (13.33), and acute atypical interstitial pneumonia ("fog fever") (5.28). Silo gas causes nitric acid formation in lungs.

13.28. Nitrate/nitrite toxicity: brown vaginal mucosa in severe methemoglobinemia (Netherlands)

13

13.29. Lead poisoning: head-pressing blind calf (Gloucester)

13.30. Iodine toxicity: dry seborrheic dermatitis in calf (Friesian)

Management: treatment with intravenous methylene blue is the specific antidote, and fluid therapy is effective in many cases.

Lead (plumbism)

Definition: acute or chronic lead poisoning results from lead deposition in various tissues, including bone, where it is in an inert form. Lead adversely affects sulfhydryl-containing enzymes and tissues rich in mitochondria, leading to cerebellar hemorrhage and edema.

Clinical signs: in lead poisoning, which remains the most commonly diagnosed cause of poisoning in cattle in the UK, the major signs of central nervous system (CNS) involvement are depression, champing of jaws, blindness, and, often, head-pressing. Some cases exhibit maniacal behavior. The 1-month-old Gloucester calf in 13.29 shows severe CNS signs. Unable to stand, its head and neck are extended to push against the brick wall. It was also blind and anorexic. Lead is a common toxicological problem in younger cattle. The source, usually environmental, is often paint from old doors, as in this calf, although crankcase oil from farm machinery, lead batteries, and contaminated feedstuffs are other sources.

Differential diagnosis: polioencephalomalacia (CCN) (9.1), listeriosis (9.11), meningitis (9.22), sudden onset of metabolic disease.

Management: individual therapy consists of calcium EDTA i.v. or s.c. for several days, plus oral magnesium sulfate to render any remaining lead unavailable as lead sulfate, and also thiamine. Note that meat withhold times in recovered cases may be several months to allow excretion of stored lead. Lead is excreted into milk.

Iodine (iodism)

Definition: excess oral intake of inorganic and organic iodine compounds.

Clinical features: common sources are ethylenediamine dihydroiodide (EDDI) in a feed additive (for footrot prevention) and potassium iodide for treatment of actinobacillosis or over-zealous dietary supplementation. Nonspecific skin changes, lacrimation, nasal discharge, hypersalivation, and a chronic cough are the usual signs. Iodism in this calf (13.30) is manifested by a dry seborrheic dermatitis primarily affecting the head and neck. Recovery followed removal of the excess element.

Differential diagnosis: dermatophilus (3.37–3.43), lice (3.20–3.24), ringworm (3.25–3.27), cutaneous lymphosarcoma.

Fluorosis

Clinical features: fluorosis usually results from the prolonged ingestion of fluorine in high-fluorine–phosphatic supplementary feeds, or fertilizers, or from herbage ingested from pastures contaminated by industrial emissions such as aluminum smelters and brick works. Deep wells are important sources of fluorine poisoning in Australia and South America. Two forms of chronic toxicity occur: osteofluorosis, and dental fluorosis which affects only erupting teeth. High intake of fluorine by adults does not cause tooth abnormalities. Dental fluorosis can be caused by as little as 20–40 ppm in diet, while skeletal fluorosis requires much higher and longer-term exposure. The absorption capacity is much higher in young animals and on high-concentrate diets, both of which predispose to toxicity. Large periosteal plaques form on long bones. 13.31 shows several enlargements that are firm and smooth to the touch on the medial aspects of the metatarsi. In 13.32 the extensive periosteal plaques, which do not involve the articular surfaces, are seen next to normal metatarsi (to the left). Cattle may become lame owing to osteoporosis, osteomalacia, and periarticular bone proliferation. Another sign of chronic disease is mottling of the temporary incisors (see 4.29). Temporary teeth can be damaged while *in utero*, the permanent dentition exposed to intoxication before their eruption.

Differential diagnosis: degenerative joint disease (7.114), aphosphorosis (7.164), selenosis (13.19), enzootic calcinosis (13.14–13.16).

13.31. Fluorosis: bone enlargements on medial aspect of metatarsi (USA)

Management: difficult in affected cattle, but oral aluminum salts and parenteral calcium are used. Prevention by altering water supply and grazing regime. Commercial defluorination of rock phosphate has made these toxic deposits safe.

Copper

Definition: excess copper ingested and accumulated over a period of time is suddenly released from its liver store, causing lipid peroxidation, intravascular hemolysis, and severe clinical signs.

Clinical features: copper toxicosis in cattle tends to be chronic, although the onset of clinical signs may be acute and associated with stress. The source may be an error of copper supplementation, or ingestion of pasture with an abnormal level of copper (from slurry or fertilizer top-dressing). The sudden onset of clinical signs of depression, weakness, thirst, and jaundice may result from a hemolytic crisis. Affected animals have dark urine due to hemoglobinuria as well as methemoglobin. The major autopsy changes include a large, friable, icteric liver and a characteristic bluish-black ("gunmetal") coloring of the kidneys (13.33). Note the color of the urine in the

13.33. Copper toxicosis: enlarged friable liver, gunmetal kidney, and dark urine (tube)

adjacent tube. Many cows have high liver copper levels but show no adverse effects. High liver and kidney values are necessary to confirm poisoning.

Differential diagnosis: calfhood leptospirosis (10.4), necrotic hepatitis (4.98), babesiosis (12.39–12.43), anaplasmosis (12.44–12.47), other causes of hemolytic anemia.

Management: individual treatment of sick cattle is usually hopeless. Ammonium molybdenate and sodium sulfate reduce the copper content of tissues and increase its fecal excretion. Symptomatic treatment, e.g., gastrointestinal sedatives, may be given. Control by eradication of plants causing phytogenous or hepatogenous copper poisoning may prove impossible, but top-dressing pastures with molybdenum at 70 g/ha or molybdenum dietary supplementation may be feasible. Dietary copper intakes are limited by legislation in the EU, with a veterinary prescription needed for compound feeds containing more than 40 ppm copper in the dry matter.

Molybdenum

Definition: molybdenum toxicity is related to copper, molybdenum, and inorganic sulfate, molybdenum and

13.32. Fluorosis: extensive periosteal plaques on metatarsal bones (USA)

13.34. Molybdenum toxicity: depigmented coat, alopecia, and periocular gray hairs (China)

13

sulfur giving rise to thiomolybdates, with which copper reacts in the rumen to produce a poorly-absorbed and insoluble complex. Toxicity usually arises from high levels of molybdenum in soil and pasture (see below).

Clinical features: molybdenum toxicosis tends to involve a relative copper deficiency. The cow from China (13.34) is thin and shows depigmentation of the normally dark coat. Note the grayish hairs around the eyes. Alopecia is present over the neck, shoulder, and withers. Note also the combination halter and nose ring used in Jiangxi Province. Many cattle with molybdenum toxicity show a persistent diarrhea, weight loss, and depigmentation of black hair also typical of the high-molybdenum "teart" pastures in parts of England.

Differential diagnosis: copper deficiency (7.167), cobalt deficiency (7.174).

Management: use of 1% copper sulfate in salt may control molybdenosis in areas where forage molybdenum exceeds 5 ppm. Higher levels of copper may be given. Use of drenching or pasture top-dressing has also been advised as preventative. Injection of copper glycinate may aid recovery in some clinical cases.

13

Appendix

AGID   agar gel immunodiffusion (test)
AI   artificial insemination
AV   atrioventricular (valve)
BEP   bovine erythropoietic porphyria
BEPP   bovine erythropoietic protoporphyria
BHM   bovine herpes mammillitis
BHV-1 (BoHV-1)   bovine herpesvirus-1
BIV   bovine immunodeficiency virus
BLV   bovine leukosis virus
BNP   bovine neonatal pancytopenia
BSE   bovine spongiform encephalopathy
BTV   bluetongue virus
BVD/MD   bovine virus diarrhea/mucosal disease
C_6-T_1   cervical 6–thoracic 1 (vertebrae)
CBPP   contagious bovine pleuropneumonia
CCN   cerebrocortical necrosis
CCP   corpus cavernosum penis
CEP   congenital erythropoietic porphyria
CF   complement fixation
CJLD   congenital joint laxity and dwarfism
CNS   central nervous system
CPK   creatine phosphokinase
CrCL   cranial cruciate ligament
CSF   cerebrospinal fluid
CVM   complex vertebral malformation
DJD   degenerative joint disease
DNA   deoxyribonucleic acid
EBL   enzootic bovine leukosis
ECF   East Coast fever
EDTA   ethylenediamine tetra-acetic acid
ELISA   enzyme-linked immunosorbent assay
FAO   Food and Agriculture Organization (of UN)
FB   foreign body
FFA   free fatty acids
FMD   foot-and-mouth disease
GDH   glutamate dehydrogenase
GGT   γ-glutamyl transferase
GI   gastro-intestinal
GnRH   gonadotrophic releasing hormone
HBS   hemorrhagic bowel syndrome
IBK   infectious bovine keratoconjunctivitis
IBR   infectious bovine rhinotracheitis
IFAT   immunofluorescent antibody test
IPVV   infectious pustular vulvovaginitis

ITEME   infectious thrombotic meningoencephalitis
i.v.   intravenous
JHS   jejunal hemorrhagic syndrome
L4   larval stage 4
L4–6   lumbar vertebrae 4–6
LDA   left displaced abomasum
LSD   lumpy-skin disease
MCF   malignant catarrhal fever
NSAID   nonsteroidal anti-inflammatory drug
nvCJD   new variant Creutzfeldt–Jakob disease
OCD   osteochondrosis dissecans
OIE   Office International des Épizooties
O-P   organophosphorus
P1   phalanx 1
P2   phalanx 2
P3   phalanx 3 (distal phalanx)
PCR   polymerase chain reaction
PDA   patent ductus arteriosus
PI-3   parainfluenza-3
PPH   pruritis-pyrexia-hemorrhagica
PTE-CVC   pulmonary thromboembolism-caudal vena caval thrombosis
PUFAs   polyunsaturated fatty acids
RDA   right displaced abomasum
RSV   respiratory syncytial virus
RVF   Rift Valley fever
SAA   serum amyloid A
SARA   subacute ruminal acidosis
SBE   sporadic bovine encephalitis
SBV   Schmallenberg virus
s.c.   subcutaneous
SCC   squamous cell carcinoma
SDH   sorbital dehydrogenase
SGOT   serum glutamic oxaloacetic transaminase
SMCO   S-methylcysteine sulfoxide
spp.   species
SuHV-1   suid herpesvirus 1
TB   tuberculosis
TEME   thrombotic meningoencephalitis
TME   thrombotic meningoencephalitis
UMD   ulcerative mammary dermatitis
UV   ultraviolet
VSD   ventricular septal defect

Index

Printed and bound by CPI Group (UK) Ltd, Croydon, CR0 4YY

08/05/2025

01864674-0001